Coping with
RHEUMATOID ARTHRITIS

Dr Judy Bury, the General Editor of this series, has worked in general practice and family planning for many years. She writes regularly on medical topics, and has a particular interest in self-help approaches to health care.

Coping with
RHEUMATOID ARTHRITIS

HEATHER UNSWORTH
Dip COT, SROT, FETC

With a Foreword by
Mrs PHIL SMITH

Chambers

Published by W & R Chambers Ltd Edinburgh

ISBN 0 550 20510 1

British Library Cataloguing in Publication Data

Unsworth, Heather
    Coping with rheumatoid arthritis.
    1. Rheumatoid arthritis
    I. Title
    362.1'96722   RC933
    ISBN 0-550-20510-1

Printed by Clark Constable, Edinburgh and London

Contents

Heather Unsworth is a Senior Occupational Therapist involved in research and training at a general hospital. Her current interests are the establishment of readily-available sources of self-help and information for the new sufferer and family; her particular concerns are with hand function and the prevention of unnecessary disability. This book has evolved as a result of a two-year research project to ascertain the needs of the new rheumatoid arthritis sufferer.

Acknowledgements

I would like to thank the following:

Dista Products Limited for sponsorship in reproducing the questionnaire and booklets for the project upon which this book was based.

The Rheumatologists of Southampton and Salisbury Health Authorities, plus the Metrology Service of East Dorset, for permission to use their patients to evaluate the book's contents.

All sufferers (and in particular Mrs Rosemary Williams) who gave freely of their time to complete questionnaires and give constructive criticism regarding the original script.

Salisbury Chiropody Department for footcare information for Chapter 8.
Mrs Marlene Clayson (Ward Sister) for Chapters 4 and 12.
Mrs Pat Grant for contributions and Chapter 13.

Miss Kathleen Fielding (District Occupational Therapist), Mrs Jean Kerley (Research Physiotherapist) and Mrs Sandra Horne (Clinical Psychologist) for advice and support.

Occupational Therapy colleagues (Miss Carole Roberts and Mrs Sue Arnold) for assistance in the initial planning stages.

Mrs Rae Hartgill and Mr John Gisby (of the Wessex Rehabilitation Association) for advice and secretarial assistance.

Heather Unsworth

Foreword

Rheumatoid arthritis (RA), one of the many rheumatic diseases, has been known to man for a long time. In the past, for those diagnosed as having this disease there has been little to offer in the way of information or advice. Patients have been told 'Of course there is no known cure' or even 'You'll have to learn to live with it' — familiar terms for many of us. Faced with trying to get by each day these words can be hard to accept and often come at a time when one is least able to understand or cope.

I've been around arthritis for 27 years one way or another, experiencing the disease both second-hand (my mother had RA) and then first-hand. In that time, through this personal knowledge and later through my close contact with other arthritis sufferers of all ages, it has become apparent that there is a very great need for information and educational material that is aimed at actually trying to help the patient understand what's in store for them, while in turn offering some facts, ideas and tips on how to come to terms and cope with the disease process of rheumatoid arthritis.

At last patients are being seen and treated as people. More and more we are able to assume some responsibility for our own bodies, illnesses, treatments and future. In order to do this successfully we need to know more about rheumatoid arthritis and what to expect from it. We need to know how the disease process develops, and learn of the medication and other treatment that is available. We need to learn of the importance of rest and conserving energy, but also of the equal importance of exercise in the management of the condition. We need to understand the reason for joint protection and skin care, and to look at ways to cope with personal hygiene and improve personal relationships. These are just some of the things that affect each of us to some degree, and if we learn to cope with these we can ensure that we make the most of ourselves and our lives.

So many publications outline the medical facts without mentioning the real problems that can be faced by each individual. These real needs and problems are looked at and discussed in this book in a clear, factual, but lighthearted way. It goes a long way towards answering the thoughts and questions that most commonly occur. It will be useful for those newly diagnosed or introduced to the disease, but will be equally helpful for those who have had the disease for some time and are still finding out how to help themselves.

The greater the knowledge and understanding we all have of rheumatoid arthritis and rheumatic disease, the greater the future prospects will be for each individual. The knowledge gained from this book will help many people to make decisions and take positive steps forward to improve their everyday lives.

With this sort of knowledge available for all to read and learn from, it must mean that the understanding, treatment and management of arthritis in the *next* 27 years can only get better !!

Mrs Phil Smith, Chairman, 35 Group, Arthritis Care.

1. Some Initial Information

Rheumatoid Arthritis

'I learnt mostly by trial and error. Why is it we always have to ask? It makes you feel that you are wasting everyone's time. Couldn't someone spare the time to explain everything, i.e. day to day living with arthritis?'

'After a clinic I forgot a lot of what I had been told because I was overwhelmed. I needed it written down.'

Rheumatoid arthritis is a disease which principally affects the joints, but it can also affect other tissues, which is why you may feel generally unwell. The disease causes inflammation of the linings of the joints, which leads to pain and eventually to changes in the bone itself — so that movement is less smooth than normal.

There are many different types of arthritis, but the term *rheumatoid* arthritis should not be confused with *osteo*-arthritis, which involves 'wear and tear' of the joints, and is a very different condition.

'My fiancé told me what the medical books said and scared me to death. As a result I got very depressed, attempted suicide and ended up with a shrink — but *still* no rheumatologist. I was 18, alone in a bedsit in an inner city with no family help or support. Only by my own efforts have I been able to learn anything — I should *not* have had to fight for it. *It is every patient's right to know how to help himself.*'

The purpose of this book is to provide information and advice for anyone with rheumatoid arthritis — or for their family. It will include information about the disease and about the treatments available, but most of all there will be information and advice on *how to help yourself* — whether you have just been diagnosed as having rheumatoid arthritis or whether you have had it for years. There are many quotes from sufferers.

What causes it?

No one really knows — although research continues to try and resolve the problem. After much study, doctors and scientists now believe that it is caused by the body becoming 'allergic' to itself so that it no longer recognises its own tissues and starts to attack them. Rheumatoid arthritis is therefore classed as an 'auto-immune disease', but it is still not known why it should happen. What *is* known, however, is that in some people certain factors, such as shock or bereavement, may trigger off the illness. These 'trigger factors' are various and, to add to the confusion, few people will have been affected by the same one. However, for every person who can pinpoint a trigger factor there will be one who cannot — such is the nature of this illness which never affects two people in the same way.

Is it infectious?

No! It cannot be passed from one person to another.

Is it inherited?

Not really. Some people inherit the tendency to get rheumatoid arthritis and it might therefore be more common in some families. However, it is the *tendency* towards the condition that is passed on, *not* the disease itself; and even if you have this tendency, you may not meet the factor that would trigger the illness in you. This is why some people who are affected can find no trace of the illness in their family history whereas others will find that several close relatives are sufferers.

Who gets rheumatoid arthritis?

It affects 1 in 50 of all adults, and women are three times more likely to be affected than men. Although the average age of onset is between 30 and 60 years of age, the disease can also affect babies, children and the elderly.

How will it affect me?

'My first major question concerned whether or not I would find myself in a wheelchair like another patient outside, but I didn't ask because of lack of knowledge as to what to ask. I did chat to another sufferer who told me that her disease started in the same way as mine and she was now confined to a wheelchair as well. This depressed me greatly. I wish now that I had received more information on drugs, diet, what and what not to do, plus how to reduce my pain. Instead I learnt by bitter experience.'

Each individual is affected differently. *No two people can be compared* and any similarity between those affected may well end with the name. The usual symptoms are pain, tenderness and swelling of the affected joints, accompanied by inflammation. You may feel tired, weak, feverish and generally off-colour, with loss of appetite and loss of weight. In most people, the initial attack soon dies down without causing much damage and you may think that you have had a severe dose of 'flu. However, further attacks are likely and are known as 'flare-ups'. It is important that treatment starts as early as possible, not just to reduce the inflammation (as your joints may have become hot and swollen) but also to start joint care (see Chapter 6). 'Flare-ups' may sometimes be related to illness, severe emotional stress, or accident, or they may come completely 'out of the blue'. Your affected joints will feel tender and stiff, especially on waking in the morning, and movement will be painful and restricted. After several attacks it is likely that your joints will become more severely affected and may become deformed. However, the severity of the attacks, their frequency and even the extent of any disability will depend upon the individual.

To give you a better idea of the varied way in which people are affected, here are some figures. Out of 20 people who have an attack of rheumatoid arthritis, 6 will have no further trouble, whilst a further 4 will have few problems, only experiencing occasional joint pains. Of the remaining 10, 6 will have active disease and some deformity, 2 will also have some deformity but may be symptom-free for long periods of time, and only 2 will eventually be confined to wheelchair or bed. In other words, half of those who have an attack of rheumatoid arthritis will have little or no further trouble, and less than one in three will be severely affected.

In later stages the disease generally becomes less active, with some people virtually being symptom-free. The degree of disability will vary greatly, from virtually none to quite severe due to damage to the joints. However advances in medical care have led to earlier diagnosis, better treatment and management, which all affect the outcome.

Early morning stiffness

Sometimes pain and stiffness are worse in the morning and it may even take you up to two hours to settle down. Be prepared for a slow start and plan your morning accordingly. Your doctor may be able to adjust your tablets so do mention any problems to him/her.

What about stress?

Some people tend to develop the disease following prolonged periods of worry or stress and others after a severe shock or illness.

Remember

No two people are affected
in the same way

What about treatment?

There are a large number of treatments available and although none can cure the arthritis, many are a great help.

Let us look first at what the *doctor* can offer.

Some people will be treated entirely by their GP whilst others will be referred to their local hospital. There may be a clinic nearby, which specialises in this form of arthritis, or you may even be sent to one away from your home area. This has nothing to do with the severity of your illness, but will depend upon where you live.

Drugs

Your doctor will decide on either one tablet or a combination of various tablets to help control your illness and relieve pain and stiffness. He/she will choose the one which is regarded as being the most suitable for you — if it doesn't suit or give any relief, then do say so, in order that the doctor can consider changing to another one. See Chapter 4 for more information about drugs.

Remember

Take your medication regularly and
as prescribed ... otherwise you will not give it a
chance to work

Surgery

There are some operations which can be a great help to sufferers from rheumatoid arthritis and much publicity is given to subjects like joint replacement. If one or more of your joints become very damaged and you find funtion increasingly difficult, then surgery may be suggested. Just when and if surgery is carried out will depend upon both you and your doctor. Surgery is not a cure, and although it can help to restore lost movement or relieve pain when a joint goes out of line, it cannot restore strength unless the weakness is caused by pain. It is for reasons such as this that not everybody can benefit from operations and your doctor may decide upon alternative measures, such as splinting (see Chapter 11).

Now let us look at some other types of treatment.

Heat treatment

A heat lamp may bring temporary relief to a painful joint, but is no real help in the long run as its benefits are short-lived. In addition, some people find that heat can actually aggravate the condition. Before buying a heat lamp, ask your doctor's advice. He/she may suggest a visit to a physiotherapist who will look at various methods of pain relief, including heat. If you use a heat lamp, it should be at least 18″ away from the joint and you should use it for about 20 minutes only (but don't forget to allow for the heating-up period). It is not always necessary to buy expensive lamps as heat pads or even a hot water bottle wrapped in a towel will have a similar effect.

Therapy

There are two kinds of therapy available to you — physiotherapy and occupational therapy. Both are concerned with relief of pain, improving or maintaining your level of function, and generally giving advice on how to cope with your disease on a day-to-day basis. The *physiotherapist* can advise on the role of exercise versus rest and how to balance the two to greatest effect. He/she can also teach you about the best ways of avoiding strain on your joints when moving and show you ways of helping relieve your pain by using either heat or cold. The *occupational therapist* will look at how you perform everyday tasks and advise on simple ways of avoiding unnecessary pain or strain. This might mean planning your day differently to save energy, altering the height of your chair if you have backache or painful knees, or even job-sharing by enlisting the help of family and friends. Contrary to what you might believe, it is *never* too early to be helped — so ask your doctor to be referred to these therapists.

'If I had had physiotherapy and occupational therapy in the early stages, perhaps I wouldn't have got as bad as this.'

Splints

Do not be surprised if your therapist wishes to make splints for you. Splints are an excellent way of resting a painful joint, whilst allowing you to continue doing activities. You might even be asked to wear one at night as this is the best way to prevent joints from going out of shape whilst you are not able to check them. Nowadays modern plastic materials mean that neat and lightweight designs can be made to measure. Your physiotherapist or occupational therapist will discuss this with you and explain what is required.

Can I do anything to help myself?

'I have had arthritis for 6 years now and am 29 years old. I know that I should have asked the doctor what I could do to prevent the arthritis from flaring up and whether diet or drink have any effect. I haven't asked because I am too nervous and don't have enough knowledge about the condition to know whether my questions are valid. I don't want to feel a fool.'

'One of the worst things about rheumatoid arthritis is feeling that you have been shelved and that you can do nothing to help yourself — that leads to depression.'

There are several things that you can do to help control the disease. Firstly, avoid getting overweight as this will put extra strain on affected joints. You should also rest when necessary and *never* try to work off pain and inflammation — despite what friends or relatives may advise. Try to recognise anything that might trigger off a flare-up and get your priorities in order — decide what you really must do and what can wait. In this way, if you are feeling a little 'under the weather', you will be able to conserve energy to plan something more important, like a special outing.

Diets

From time to time great publicity is given to special diets but after much study doctors can still find no reason to think that they are either the cause or the cure for arthritis. It is essential that you stick to a good balanced diet which makes you neither over- or underweight. At all times be sensible, as it is vital that you eat sufficient of the essential nutrients to help your body to cope with everyday demands. However, if you do suspect that your diet may be at fault, and a certain food is making your symptoms worse, then do mention it to your doctor. He/she may suggest that you avoid the suspect food and be referred to a dietician for further advice.

Joint Care

Follow the guidelines on why joint care is important and on looking after your joints. Only *you* can do this and it is equally as important as taking your tablets because your joints when inflamed need a little extra care.

Interests

Don't give up your interests and hobbies, continue them wherever practicable, if necessary in moderation, or find new ones.

There are four golden rules that you can adopt:
Pain … try to avoid it;

Pacing and planning ... don't take on more than you can cope with, so plan ahead;

Protection ... don't subject your joints to unnecessary stress;

Learn to recognise your body signals and you will know just how far to go before it complains!

Some questions answered

'What is best, exercise or rest?' *Both* — in moderation! Too much exercise or heavy work may cause damage to your joints, but a moderate amount will help to keep them supple. Similarly there are times when you will want to rest a joint and times when you find too much sitting or lying makes you feel stiff.

**Everyone must find their own balance
between doing too much and doing too little**

'What is best, heat or cold?' Some people find that heat is beneficial and that cold, damp weather makes them feel worse. If you are affected this way, start the day with either a warm bath or shower. Even soaking your hands in a bowl of warm water will help. On the other hand some people find that they are worse in heat and soaking hands in cold water is the answer. Whichever temperature suits you best, adjust your home atmosphere accordingly.

You may find it helpful to buy a Thermos camping pack as this retains either heat or cold for up to two hours. The 'liquid' types are most successful as they can be applied direct to the joint. Similarly, a pack of frozen peas wrapped in a towel makes a useful ice pack.

Old wives' tales

'Copper bracelets ease arthritis.' There is no evidence that copper jewellery will help, but it can certainly do no harm.

'Hard work never hurt anyone.' Well-meaning friends and relatives may advise you to overcome your pain by 'working it off', but this is probably the worst thing that you can do!

Inflamed, painful joints need rest, not hard work; in fact hard work may even harm them. In the same way that you would go to bed with a dose of 'flu, so you should rest with a flare-up.

'Cold, damp weather causes arthritis.' Although you may feel more aches and stiffness, it is not the cause of arthritis. In fact, some people actually feel better in colder weather.

'If I had received information 7 years ago when first diagnosed, I would have been saved a lot of pain and worry instead of finding out the hard way. General information should be available, not just for the sufferer, but also for the family and general public. All too often arthritics are accused of being 'bloody-minded' when sitting on bus seats that OAPs regard as their own or when we say that we cannot lift heavy shopping or help others. Sometimes other people just do not realise the severe pain that we go through and either nag or bury their head in the sand.'

'To be forewarned is to be forearmed! Treatment and medication with little in the way of explanation almost cancels its usefulness. It is essential to know what movements to avoid to minimise the worst effects of RA. Most people can cope with a situation if given the facts, but my biggest problem initially was feeling guilty and thinking that as a mother and wife I had let the family down. This depression and frustration was very difficult to handle as I had led a very active life. I had outbursts of bitter anger — which luckily my family understood. A large percentage of coping is understanding and the support of family and friends. I know that I made life pretty awful at times for my family. However, 25 years later, I would advise any new sufferer that a positive attitude is most important — and the ability to live one day at a time will get you through.'

2. Posture: Resting, Working, and Driving Positions

It is always important to think about good *posture* but it becomes more so if you are affected by an arthritic condition. It is a common mistake to try to compensate by shifting the weight off painful joints and on to other less painful ones. This not only has the effect of putting more stress on the joint but also causes unnecessary muscle strain and contributes significantly towards deformities.

Your therapist will advise you on all aspects of standing, sitting, lying and working positions, but here are some suggestions to supplement what you are told.

Standing

Stand upright with your head held up.

Keep your back straight, shoulders relaxed, tummy and bottom tucked in.

Stand firmly on both feet, letting them take the weight equally.

Wear comfortable, supportive shoes with insoles if necessary.

Avoid standing for long periods of time. When possible use a stool, perching stool or shooting stick.

Sitting

Avoid soft or low chairs. The correct height chair should be high enough to get on and off with the least stress.

Choose a seat with a good back support.

Upholstery should be supportive but comfortable.

Arm rests and a head rest provide more support.

A foot rest may help but otherwise the feet should be placed flat on the floor.

Change positions frequently to avoid stiffness in the joints.

Lying

Your *bed* should be a good height to prevent strain on the knees and hips when getting in and out; if it sags, fit a board under the mattress.

The *mattress* itself should be firm so that it provides good support and is easier to get up from.

If you find *bedclothes* too heavy, a duvet or continental quilt will help.

A *small pillow* will be most comfortable for your neck; in any case, avoid using more than one pillow. A useful guideline as to the correct pillow height is that the head should not be pushed forwards. A useful tip is to make a 'butterfly' pillow. This gives good support but is comfortable. A soft scarf, length of bandage or old stocking can be used to tie the pillow in the middle.

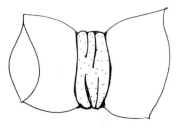

Butterfly Pillow

Never put a pillow beneath the knees as this will encourage them to become fixed in a bent position!

If you cannot bear bedclothes on your feet, borrow a bed cradle from the Red Cross or make your own from a cardboard box or fireguard.

Working position

As for sitting — but make sure that your work is also at the *right height* to match your chair! Too high a chair will cause back and neck ache because you are having to lean forward and look down. If your chair will not go lower, *raise the height* of your table or desk with blocks. Working at an inclined desk or desk lectern will take the strain off your back and neck by making your work posture more upright.

Small lumbar support cushions which fit snugly into the 'small' of your back may also be helpful and can be purchased through many of the larger chemist's shops.

Use collar or wrist supports if recommended by your therapist or doctor.

A telephone receiver rest may also be useful, especially if the shoulders or elbows are painful — contact British Telecom or a local aids centre for advice on what is available.

Driving

Exercise moderation with your driving — keep distances to a sensible length depending upon your condition. On good days *beware* — don't overtax yourself or you will be overtired later.

If you are having difficulty with your car seat, door handles or controls, ask to be referred to an occupational therapist, who will show you where to try out various modifications and levers that are available on the market. Your local garage may also help you by adapting difficult controls, such as the handbrake, if you are troubled by weakness.

Having small adaptations done is not giving in

Why struggle when help is available? Your energy will be sapped and your painful joints more stressed if you don't seek advice. If you are not able to contact an occupational therapist, the British School of Motoring may help.

Point to note: if you wear a collar for driving, or have any alterations done to your car, don't forget to inform your insurance company.

Remember

Do not sit in one position for too long —
get up and move about

3. Resting, Planning and Energy Conservation

Rest

'I am 64 years old and have had RA for the past 12 years. Now that I am older, I wish that I had been told how important rest is and not to keep pushing myself so hard.'

Rest of an inflamed joint is an important principle in the treatment of rheumatoid arthritis — but this often seems puzzling when morning stiffness improves with exercise. People are afraid that they will 'seize up' if they do not exercise *but* it is the joints that are used *most often* that are *most inflamed*.

As exercise (in moderation) is essential, so also is rest — although the amount will vary from person to person. You must learn to find your *own* balance between rest and exercise.

Is it a treatment?

Rest is as important as taking your medicine. If your doctor feels that it may help — he/she might arrange for you to be admitted to hospital *for a complete rest*.

Rest may be the most difficult part of the whole treatment programme to follow, especially if you are a busy housewife with young children or a person in full-time employment ... *but you must try*.

What is meant by rest?

Rest can vary from reducing an activity which over-uses a joint, to complete *bed* rest. There are several stages in between.

It may be helpful to change to lighter work or spend *1-2 hours* resting on the bed *each* day.

Try different ways, to help *you* decide what is best for *you*. Resting on a bed is generally more beneficial than sitting in a chair.

Resting is not giving-in

Your body will *need* more rest when you have a flare-up. Relaxation requires skill and practice.

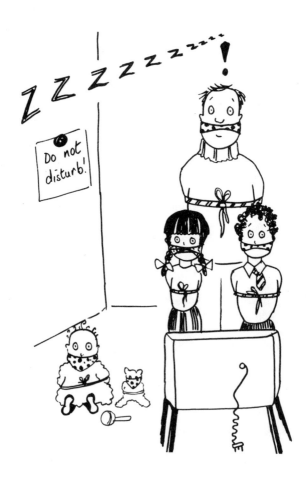

Planning and Energy Conservation

Plan your work ahead

It can often help to write out a plan for your days to make sure that you make time for the things that you need to do. Include a list of all activities, for example:

work .... social .... exercise .... rest

Assemble your family group if you can and discuss your timetable with them. Explain to them why you are doing this — and about the importance of energy conservation and rest in the treatment of rheumatoid arthritis. Discuss with them the following:

Can the job be eliminated?

Are there some jobs that don't need to be done at all or could be done by somebody else — either by another member of the family or by paying someone?

e.g.	ironing sheets	cleaning car
	laundry	gardening
	preparing vegetables	fixing the car
	drying dishes	'do it yourself' tasks.

Which members of the family can help most?

Go through everything that needs to be done and work out who can do what — perhaps on a rota.

e.g.	meal preparation	lifting
	shopping	cutting the hedge
	making beds	cleaning the car
	washing-up	mending the car
	washing/ironing	painting and decorating/DIY
	cleaning and housework	mowing the lawn.

Then divide the list into heavy and light jobs, distribute them evenly throughout the week — remembering that heavy jobs can be broken down into smaller parts.

Can the job be made more simple?

Think about the jobs that you *have* to do — can you organise them better?

e.g.   Cook and serve from the same dish.

Gather dirty laundry at the same time as making beds and putting clothes away.

Gather all most commonly used items into one area to save trips.

Measure all dry ingredients before starting to cook. This will save washing dishes.

'Your biggest ally could be your husband. I am lucky enough to have an understanding and domesticated husband who cheerfully undertook all the heavy chores in the early days, such as hoovering, shopping and ironing. After a full day's work he would come in and make a cup of tea and give me a short spell with my feet up, recuperating from the demands of the children, and this I found invaluable and it enabled me to continue with the supper etc. afterwards. If this is not possible then you *must* at least train both your husband and the rest of the family to not hinder. This sounds odd, but you will be so grateful for the energy spared when you have taught them all to put everything away as they use it, collect their dirty washing and put it in the right place, not to leave tools, toys etc. all over the floor where you can trip and do yourself an injury. My maxim has become "If you cannot help, then please do not hinder." Other children must be taught to do the same and encouraged to help as much as possible. In the darkest days my 9-year-old would give me half-an-hour after school each day for any special tasks I needed done. He became very good at chopping vegetables and tasks that I found difficult. He was also very good at fetching and carrying for the baby and entertaining him for a short while so that I could sit down or put my feet up for 10 minutes if things got on top of me. You can supervise just as well sitting down!'

'I am so grateful for good friends and neighbours. If you do not have any, you are going to miss out. But are you sure you have none? People I barely knew began to arrive on my doorstep asking to be allowed to shop, cook, work or take the baby out. I was overwhelmed by kindness and I must admit my pride resented it. How hard it is to sit and watch your friend scrub your kitchen floor. I have now learned to be generous. By this I mean that I have discovered that people *want* to help. They like to feel needed in helping. One neighbour was pushing my trolley round Sainsbury's for me as I recited my list while she reached for the items, and I mentioned to her how onerous she must find this.

"Oh no," she said, "you so enjoy being taken to the shops instead of just sending someone that I am looking at Sainsbury's with different eyes and really enjoying myself." I progressed from someone really embarrassed at any help to someone who would, if necessary, ring up one of the numbers on my growing list of helpers and ask for assistance. People dropped in whenever they were passing — not to stay but to see if I was O.K. and all would respond to frantic hand-waving from the window if I needed help with a nappy! Do not think you can do nothing for them in return. You may be unable to do anything very physical but you can always give them what everyone wants — a listening ear for their troubles and time to talk. Most able-bodied people are very short of that commodity called time.'

'If you are severely limited, you have a large family and insufficient friends and relations to rally round, you may need to resort to paid help. This will depend on your financial position and there are not many people able to afford full-time nannies. However, you can consider a cleaner once a week to do "the heavy" or if you are really desperate a nursery or childminder perhaps one or two half days. We solved the problem by joining in the au pair system.'

'Every labour-saving device you can possibly afford you need. A washing-machine is essential or somebody to visit the launderette. Our greatest help was a microwave cooker. It means no more working with heavy saucepans or hot heavy dishes from the oven. Nothing burns on, so the dishes are easy to clean. The handles do not get hot, and you cannot burn yourself on the oven.'

'If you do not have a microwave you need lightweight saucepans, easy recipes and should either give up peeling vegetables or enrol someone to do it for you. We found someone happy to batch-bake for the freezer at low cost for a while.'

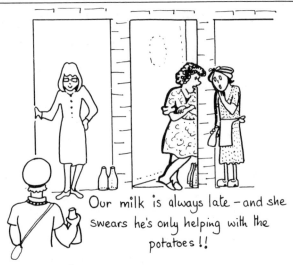

Our milk is always late – and she swears he's only helping with the potatoes !!

Your occupation

Apply the same planning principles to your occupation:

Can any part of your job be eliminated?

Can any part of your job be given to somebody else?

Can any part of your job be simplified by planning ahead?

Then think of ways to organise your job to fit in with your lifestyle.

Consider whether any part of your job can be divided into heavy and light tasks — and evenly spread throughout the week.

Would your employer allow you to work flexi-hours?

Could you extend your lunch break so that you can rest, and work a slightly longer day?

Could you start work later on the days that you have early morning joint stiffness?

Would you allow a member of your family to dress you or take you to work — to help you save energy for your job?

This will be a basic guide for you *but* your timetable must be adaptable to include social and recreational activities *and* allow for the fluctuating behaviour of the disease.

'Take the good days and be thankful, but do not overdo things when you feel better — which is a temptation — especially if you have an active mind (the voice of experience!).'

'One word of warning — do nothing and you will become depressed; do too much and you will pay for it in terms of aching joints and exhaustion. Pick and choose your invitations, and conserve energy by doing only what you really want to do. After all, you have a good excuse!'

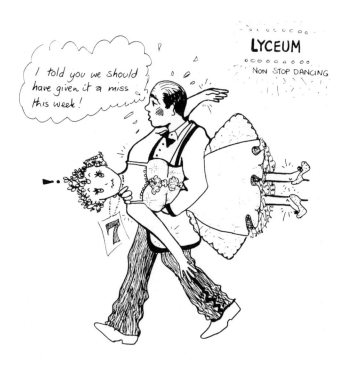

Remember
Always start the job with the understanding
that you can stop for a rest

4. Know Your Medication

'I would have liked more information about side effects of drugs as I found it worrying to be suddenly taking so many medicines.'

There is a wide range of medication for the treatment of rheumatoid arthritis and these are divided into groups, based on the way each works. Each medication will have more than one name, one being a trade name and the other its proper drug name. You may be confused by this so check with your doctor or pharmacist if you are concerned.

Relief of pain (Analgesics)

The preparations most commonly used to relieve pain are:—
    aspirin (Aspro, Disprin) (there are many varieties available)
    paracetamol (Panadol)
    codeine
    dihydrocodeine (DF 118)
Many pain-relieving tablets bought over the counter in chemists' shops contain mixtures of any of these drugs mentioned.
Always read the instructions on the bottle or package carefully.
Some pain-relieving drugs, e.g. paracetamol, may cause constipation.
If you are not sure when it is best to take your pain-relieving tablets, follow these simple rules:—

Never let your pain become unbearable. It is easier to prevent pain getting bad than to relieve it when it is already bad.

Follow the instructions given on the label on the bottle, such as:

TWO Tablets every 4 - 6 hours

You can use your pain-relieving tablets to control pain in advance. For example, if your joints are particularly painful in the mornings, it may help you if you take your tablets half an hour before getting out of bed. Set your alarm clock that much earlier; it may well be worth it.

Remember

It is easier to prevent pain than to lessen it
once it is there

Do not take more than is stated on the bottle. If you find that the prescribed number of tablets is not sufficient to control your pain, then make an appointment to see your doctor. If you are having a good day with little pain, it is perfectly in order to reduce the number of pain-relieving tablets you take, for example one tablet every 4 - 6 hours, instead of the stated two.

Some medicines should be taken on an empty stomach and some only with food, e.g. aspirin (see below). If you are unsure, do check with your doctor or pharmacist. In any case, do take tablets whilst sitting up, to prevent them from sticking in your throat. If you need food with your early morning medicine, have at your bedside a flask filled with milk, plus some plain biscuits.

Reduction of inflammation (Anti-inflammatories)

This group of quick-acting medicines are those which reduce inflammation and swelling in the joints whilst also relieving pain. There are many different ones available, although aspirin is most widely used because of its ability to effectively relieve pain as well as reduce inflammation and swelling.

Aspirin may cause buzzing in the ears or indigestion, when taken in large doses. *You should always take aspirin with food.* If you experience a buzzing sensation in the ears or indigestion you should consult your doctor, who may reduce the dosage. If aspirin is part of your medication, check that anything you buy (e.g. for headache or cough) does not also contain aspirin. Read the small print carefully and ask your doctor or pharmacist if in doubt.

The best dose of aspirin for you is one which relieves pain and stiffness as much as possible but does not cause buzzing in the ears or indigestion.

There are many other types of medication which help to reduce inflammation and swelling. They come in various forms; tablets or capsules, liquid or powder preparations, or as suppositories. Your doctor will decide which is the most suitable one for you. He or she will explain to you how often and when to take them.

As there are so many anti-inflammatory drugs available and still being developed, it is not possible to list them all, but here are a few:—

> naproxen (Naprosyn)
> indomethacin (Indocid)
> ibuprofen (Brufen)
> piroxican (Feldene)
> diclofenac (Voltarol)

Suppositories are inserted into the back passage (anus) each night when you go to bed. Ask your doctor or nurse to teach you how to use them.

If you are on any of these medicines, you must take them regularly, as prescribed by your doctor. Do not miss out any doses even though you are feeling well, as these drugs are not like pain-killers — they have a different action and different intention.

As with pain-relieving tablets, those to reduce inflammation must be taken with food. Any symptoms such as nausea, dizziness or skin rashes should be reported to your doctor or district nurse, as should headaches or lightheadedness.

Anti-inflammatories are sometimes referred to as Non-Steroidal Anti-Inflammatory Drugs (NSAIDs), which is to distinguish them from a different group known as 'steroids', which will be discussed later.

Other drug therapies (Anti-rheumatic drugs)

Drugs of this group are slow-acting and used to help prevent any further damage to your joint. They may be used if the previously described two groups are unsuccessful and X-ray examination reveals some joint damage. Two of these drugs are:

sodium auriothiomalate — known as gold (Myocrisin)
D-penicillamine (Distamine)

These drugs have similar actions in their ability to suppress both the disease and its progress. However, despite similar actions and side-effects, these two drugs are prepared and administered in quite different ways.

How gold is administered

Gold is given once weekly by injection, starting with a small test dose of 10mg or less. If no reaction such as a skin rash occurs, the dose may be increased to 20-50 mg weekly. After some months, the frequency of injection may be reduced to once per fortnight or even monthly depending on how good the response is. Sometimes your doctor may decide to vary the frequency of injection from monthly to weekly again.

How long will I need it? You will not have a course of gold. If you have no side-effects with this drug it will be given for a long period of up to two years and then may be gradually reduced over a further two years. If gold is stopped, there is a risk of the symptoms of joint pains and swelling returning.

Unlike some medicines, it does not matter too much if you miss an occasional dose of gold, e.g. if you are away.

Gold is a very effective drug for the treatment of rheumatoid arthritis. About one third of patients get back to nearly normal and another one third are much improved. However, the remaining third do not benefit, or have to stop taking the drug because of reactions.

Penicillamine

Penicillamine is given in tablet form, usually once daily. It has one major difference from other drugs — it is best taken on an empty stomach because it will then be absorbed into the body more effectively. Take it either in the early morning or mid-morning with a cup of coffee or tea. The presence of iron will also delay the absorption of penicillamine so, if you are also on a course of iron tablets, take these at bedtime.

Remember

When you first start taking these drugs you will not notice any change in your joints: the amount has to build up gradually in your body

It may take 2-3 months before you feel any benefit.

Side effects of gold and penicillamine

If you are on either of these two drugs, very occasionally an allergic skin reaction may occur in the form of a rash, which can be localised or widespread. No more gold or penicillamine should be taken and you should see your doctor. Other side-effects which you may get are indigestion, dizziness, small mouth ulcers, a sore throat or a metallic taste in your mouth.

Blood and urine tests. You will be having blood tests to ensure that gold and penicillamine produce no adverse effects on your blood. The test will also show your doctor whether the disease is being kept under control.

To check that your kidneys do not become affected, weekly urine tests will be carried out by your nurse, before your gold injection. If you take penicillamine you will be given a kit to enable you to do your own weekly urine tests to look for traces of protein which can be an early sign of effects on your kidneys.

If you receive either of these two drugs, you will be given a *record card* which will be filled in regularly by your doctor or nurse; any changes in your symptoms or reactions will be noted.

Hydroxychloroquine (Plaquenil)

This is another useful drug that may be suitable to your needs and rarely causes any problems. However, you will be asked to attend at an eye hospital for regular check-ups as this drug sometimes causes eye irritation.

Cyclophosphamide (Endoxana) and azathioprine (Imuran)

These drugs can be useful in the management of rheumatoid arthritis but have to be monitored very strictly due to the risk of toxic side-effects (such as skin rashes or alterations in the white cell blood count). It is because of these side-effects that these drugs are not as commonly used as others already mentioned.

Steroids (Cortisone)

Steroids or Cortisone are names given to a group of drugs which are a stronger version of a substance called cortisol, which is present in all our bodies and suppresses inflammation better than other drugs. Doctors are reluctant to prescribe steroids (because of possible side-effects) other than for short courses which may be in tablet form or as an injection into either muscle or joint. However, if for a particular reason you have to be on steroids for a period, you should observe the following rules:

Never be tempted to take more of this drug than is written on your prescription.

If your doctor decides to stop or reduce this drug, he or she will do so very gradually over a long period, so that your body can adjust and start producing its own cortisol again. (While you are on steroids, your body stops producing its own cortisol altogether.)

If during the period of reducing the dose of Cortisone you feel weak and lose your appetite, you should consult your doctor immediately. It may be due to lack of cortisol produced by your body.

When taking this drug, watch your weight carefully, as you may put on weight.

You will also find that you bruise more easily, so take care not to knock yourself.

The taking of this drug over a long period may also mask any other infection, so be aware.

You will be given a blue card with a record of the dose of steroid you are on. Any subsequent changes should be entered. Always carry this card with you; for example if you need to see a doctor when on holiday, he will need to know about your steroids.

It is important that you tell any doctor attending you that you are on steroids. For example, if you have an infection or need an operation, it may be necessary to raise the dose of steroids for a short time.

Finally, *never* stop taking this drug suddenly as this would leave you without steroids before your body has started making its own cortisol again. This would result in your becoming very ill. If for any reason you are sick and unable to take your tablets, you should call in your doctor who will give you an injection of Cortisone if necessary. *This rule applies to all steroids.*

Remember

No two people react to drugs in the same way!

General information

Always make sure your medicines are stored in a safe place out of the reach of children and preferably in a locked cupboard.

Never mix two or more different types of tablet in one container; always keep them in the original container supplied by your chemist.

If you have difficulty in opening the new standard safety bottles but can manage ordinary screw tops, ask your chemist to supply them instead.

Try to learn the names of your various tablets. Better still, make a personal treatment record — write down your drugs in a little book and note any side effects and changes in your medication regime — it is important, and it will help your doctor in planning your treatment.

Some out-patients departments give out their own information sheets about the drugs you are currently taking, which will help you to understand about your treatment, how it works, and what to look out for.

Remember

Only the most widely known forms of medication
have been described here; there are other drugs in use
and new ones are being developed all the time.
The guidelines which have been given are only basic
ones — to help you to understand your medication
régime more fully.

How to make a personal treatment record

To make your own treatment record, you should start a little book and note the following:—

1. The *date* when your diagnosis was confirmed.
2. The *dates* and *duration* of any 'flare-ups' that occur.
3. All *medication*, its *reactions* and when it is *changed* by your doctor.

You may decide to keep your record under specific headings and the following may be a guideline for you:—

Flare-up Started	Flare-up Ended	Medication	Reactions	Date	Other Treatments	Reaction

Can you answer all these questions?

1   Name your pain-relieving tablet.

2   When should you be taking your pain-relieving tablet?

3   May you miss taking your pain-relieving tablets, if you feel you do not need them?

4   Should you take your anti-inflammatory drugs all the time?

5   Should you take all your tablets on an empty stomach or with food?

6   Do gold and penicillamine work quickly or do a few months elapse before you notice any benefit?

7   Do you keep a booklet if you are on gold or penicillamine?

8   When should you take penicillamine?

   a   early morning before breakfast?

   b   at coffee time?

   c   with iron tablets?

9   Can you stop taking steroids suddenly?

10   Can your dose of steroids be reduced quickly?

11   Do you understand all your tablets and know how you should take them?

12   Do you need more help to understand your tablets and medicines and what action they perform?

   If the answer to question 12 is Yes, then see your doctor.

5. Exercise

'With hindsight, I wished I had known what to do to keep mobile. One person tells you to rest, another to exercise — I felt very confused.'

Rest is important but so also is a little exercise.

With the exception of the most acutely inflamed areas, all joints should be put through their fullest range of movement each day. It is difficult to say just how many exercises should be done in each session as you will be influenced by the way in which the joints respond.

'I found exercising very confusing as I didn't know which ones to do or how many.'

Start with the mildest type of exercise and *carefully check the effect on the joint*. At the *first sign* of increased swelling, heat, stiffness or pain, *reduce* the amount of exercise. Try again next day.

A good general rule of thumb is:

Start gently (1-3 times through each exercise).

Build up gradually (3-5 times through each exercise).

At the first sign of trouble — *stop* and review the situation.

Exercise should *never* be too strenuous or too extreme. A five-mile hike or weight training are *not* appropriate. Don't let others advise you — discuss it with your doctor or therapist.

Remember the golden rules

Balance rest with exercise
Listen to your body
Little and often

Eventually you will learn to understand your body's signals and know just how much to do and *when to rest*.

Exercise can be described as either passive or active. In *passive* exercise you do not use your own muscles but let the joint be moved through its range either by another person or your other limb. In *active* exercise you use your own muscles.

Exercise has three important functions:

to maintain or improve muscle power around the joints;

to maintain or improve the range of movement of a joint;

to help achieve a functional target or a useful goal (e.g. climbing stairs, getting out of a chair, etc).

Remember

Several short periods of exercise a day are better than one prolonged session.

Don't do all the exercises at one time.

Fit them in with your daily timetable — if you find this difficult, concentrate on several different exercises each day alternately.

(But always ensure that you are not losing movement because of this.)

A useful tip

In the same way that some people find that either heat or cold when applied to a joint is extremely soothing, so some find that it may often ease movement. If this applies to you, then try a hot or cold bath/shower each morning, to help counteract your early morning stiffness and prepare your joints for any exercise.

Daily Exercise Programme

Body exercises

Sit comfortably in a chair. Drop your head forward so that it touches your chest. Gradually lean forwards and down towards your knees. Slowly straighten up, don't unwind your head until last. Time your breathing to fit in with this.

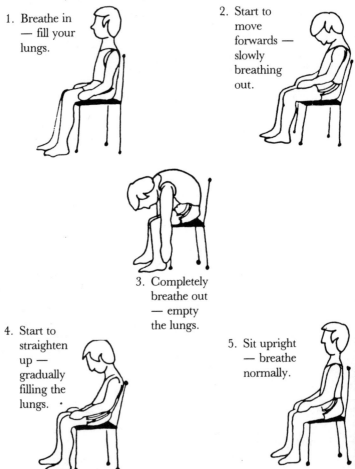

1. Breathe in — fill your lungs.

2. Start to move forwards — slowly breathing out.

3. Completely breathe out — empty the lungs.

4. Start to straighten up — gradually filling the lungs.

5. Sit upright — breathe normally.

Repeat this exercise three times.

Neck exercises

These exercises should be done *standing* with your head back against a wall or *sitting* with your head back against a high-backed chair or *lying* with a pillow.

Standing

Press your head
against the support
but keep your chin in.

Sitting

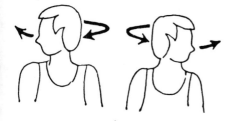

1. Bend your head to the side — right ear to shoulder — left ear to shoulder.

2. Turn your head slowly — look over one shoulder, then the other.

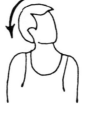
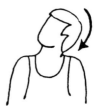

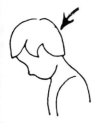
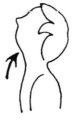

3. Drop your head gently forwards; change — and look up.

31

Shoulder and elbow exercises

Each of these exercises should be repeated three times.

Sitting

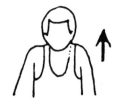

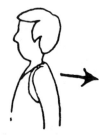

1. Shrug your shoulders up to your ears — then lower slowly.

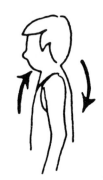

2. Pull your shoulders back, hold, and relax.

3. Circle your shoulders up, back and down.

Standing

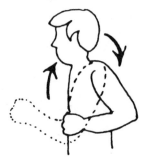

1. Bend your elbows and circle them.

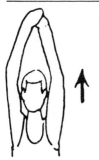

2. Hands together, stretch your arms up.

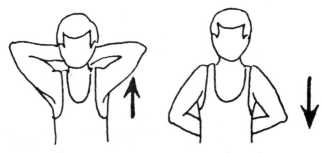

3. Place your hands behind your head and then behind your back.

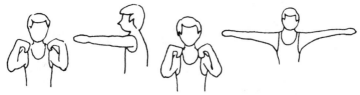

4. Touch your shoulders with your finger tips, stretch your arms forwards: touch your shoulders with finger tips, stretch your arms sideways.

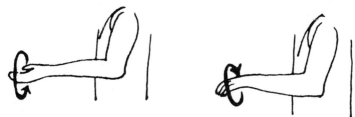

5. Holding your elbows into your waist, turn your palms up and then down.

33

Wrist and hand exercises

Sit comfortably with your forearms resting either on a table or chair arm. Alternatively support the elbow with your other hand.

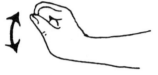

1. Bend the fingers as in a fist, but keep your fingers in a relaxed position. Move the wrist up, then down.

2. Keep the fingers bent and circle the wrist, first one way, then the other.

3. Make a fist, tighten then relax.

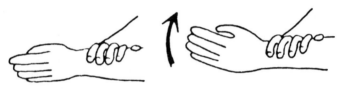

4. Straighten your fingers, place the side of the hand down on to a table or chair arm. Place your other hand on the forearm to stop it from moving. Move the hand from the wrist towards the thumb and back to the middle position. (*Never move towards the little finger*).

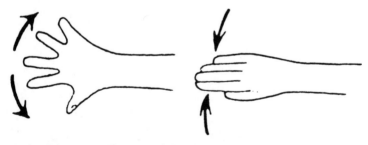

5. Straighten your fingers and thumb, span them as widely as you can, and then close them together.

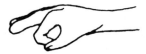 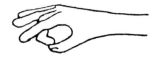

6. Touch the tip of each finger in turn with the thumb.

7. Touch the base of the little finger with the thumb.

8. Drum the fingers gently on the table (as in playing the piano).

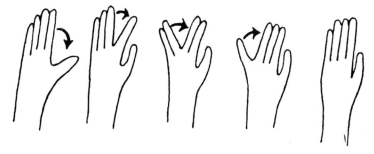

9. 'Walk' the fingers on the table *towards* the thumb.

Hip and knee exercises

Repeat this exercise three times. Lie on your back on the bed, with one pillow under your head and neck.

1. Tighten your tummy and seat muscles — hold for a count of 5 seconds then relax.

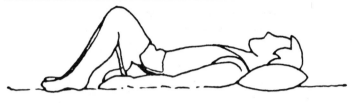

2. Bend your knees up.

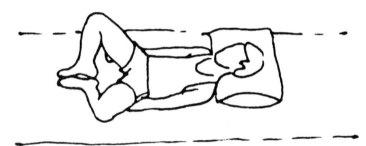

3. Part your knees, spread your legs as wide as possible (still keeping the knees bent) and close together again.

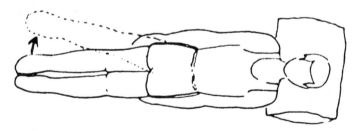

4. Straighten each leg in turn and still lying flat, lift one leg off the bed and out to the side. Bring the leg back again. Repeat the exercise with the other leg.

Exercises for the thigh muscle

There are two ways of doing these, either sitting or lying.

Lying

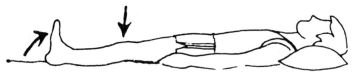

Pull up your feet, tighten your thigh muscles hard (to brace the knee) — hold for a count of 5 seconds and relax.

Sitting

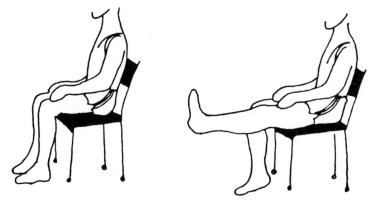

Sit with your feet flat on the ground. Straighten one leg out in front of you and then slowly bend it again. Repeat with the other leg.

Foot and ankle exercises

Lying ... on a bed with your legs outstretched:—

1. Curl your toes as tightly as you can, then uncurl them and relax.

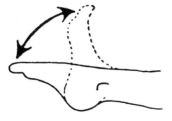

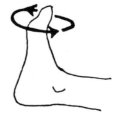

2. Pull your feet up then down.

3. Circle your feet around.

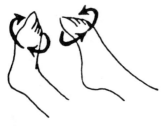

4. Turn your feet in, then out.

Stand ... using a chair back for support.

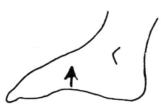

1. Press down your toes and shorten your foot by pulling up the arch on the inside of the foot.

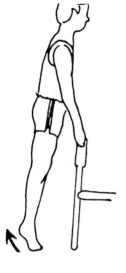

2. Raise your heels and go into tip toe position. Lower slowly.

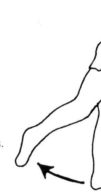

3. Then lift one leg straight and backwards. Repeat with the other leg.

Remember

These exercises are only to help keep you from becoming too stiff, not to make you 'olympic' fit, *so don't overdo them*! The purpose of any exercise is to put each joint through its own natural movements and not to subject it to any abnormal strains or contortions. You should therefore be able to tell daily if your range of movement and degree of pain are worsening or improving.

Be sensible — go carefully and pace yourself — if three times is too much, do the exercises only once or twice per day.

6. Why Joint Care is Important

The aim of this chapter is to advise you on how you can use your joints without subjecting them to the unnecessary strain that contributes towards joint deformity.

Whilst your joints are inflamed you will have to think carefully about the stresses that you subject them to. This *does not* mean giving up altogether — just re-thinking the way that you perform a function or the number of times that you do it. If the activity is a very heavy one, you may decide to avoid it altogether until your joints have settled down.

Do's and don'ts

Do think carefully each time you use your joints.

Don't think that you must do the job because it is good for you to push yourself. You *cannot* work off pain and inflammation.

Do start a job with the understanding that you can stop for a rest, stop altogether, or at least get help.

Don't get involved in lengthy jobs that tax you beyond your endurance and leave you exhausted.

Do take adequate rest. Balance your work and rest periods sensibly, to suit your *own* needs not the family's.

Remember

Today's over-enthusiasm is tomorrow's 'OUCH'!

Use your energy sensibly and keep a little in reserve.

Use your joints sensibly and think about them.

Joint Care

To help you to understand how deformity occurs and why joint care is so important, a little knowledge of the anatomy of your joints is necessary.

Joints vary depending upon the particular function that they have to perform. For example, some joints such as the hands and shoulders need to be extremely mobile with a large range of movement. Other joints such as the hips and knees bear a lot of weight and therefore need to be very stable as well as mobile.

The lining of the joints is called the synovium, so that when you hear your doctor referring to synovial tissue or synovial joints, then you will know that he/she is referring to these mobile joints. A typical synovial joint looks like this: —

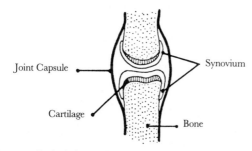

Common areas of pain, inflammation and swelling in the hand are as follows: —

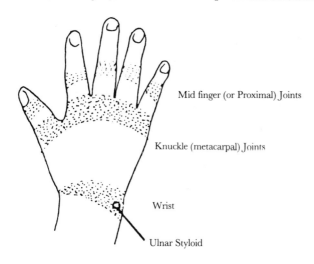

41

Laxity or slackness of the ligaments around the joints often permits more movement than normal. When this happens, sometimes the joints stay in these abnormal positions and cannot return to normal.

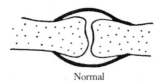

Normal

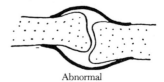

Abnormal

When this happens to the knuckles, it gives them their prominent bony look. Medically, this condition is called *subluxation*, which basically means 'out-of-joint'.

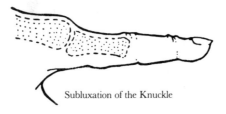

Subluxation of the Knuckle

Where the bones are no longer in contact at a joint, it is not subluxation but *dislocation*: —

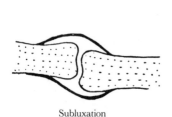

Subluxation

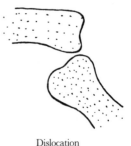

Dislocation

Due to this *laxity* of the ligaments surrounding the joints, it is not wise to put *unnecessary* pressure on the joints, especially when they are inflamed and at risk.

For this reason, you should not get up from a chair by pushing down on the knuckles and thumb.

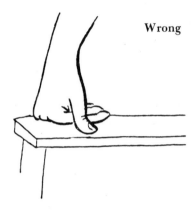

Wrong

You may hear the term *ulnar drift*. This is when the fingers are no longer in a straight line with the hand.

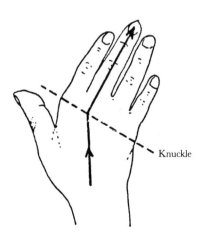

Knuckle

Ulnar drift happens because the laxity of the ligaments has allowed the knuckles to move sideways.

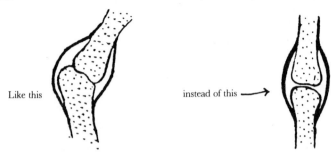

Like this   instead of this ⟶

Ulnar drift is usually seen when the wrist has also been affected. The wrist bones are known as the keystone to the hand and if the joint goes out of line, then the fingers become angled to enable them to come back into line with the forearm. This is aptly described as the *Z* or *zig-zag* deformity.

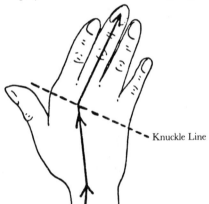

← Knuckle Line

You should now understand why you are discouraged from certain activities which put extra stress on these joints, for example pushing up from a bed, or chair, like this:

Wrong

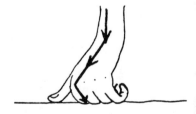

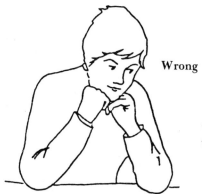

Wrong

or leaning the chin on
the fingers. like this:

For other activities which encourage deformity by placing
stress on joints — in an abnormal position — see the
remainder of this chapter.

Certain types of grip also present a risk:

1. Tight or prolonged pinch or grip } as in carrying heavy cases/bags
2. Static grip ....
3. Static grip .... as in knitting

The reasons why prolonged pinch or grip increase the deformity
risk at the knuckles is illustrated below:—

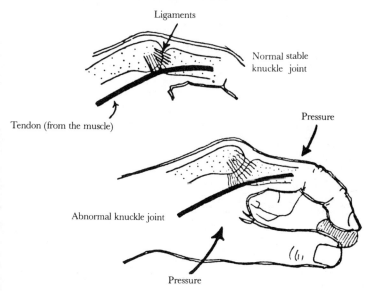

Ligaments

Normal stable
knuckle joint

Tendon (from the muscle)

Pressure

Abnormal knuckle joint

Pressure

45

The pressure caused by pinch or prolonged grip tends to pull the knuckle 'out-of-joint'. To help prevent this, only do these activities in small doses or avoid them if at all possible. However, there is a very easy way of taking the strain off your knuckles and that is to *enlarge* the handle or object that you have to grip. Look at the next two diagrams, and observe the difference in the angle (solid black line) between gripping the large and the small object.

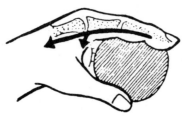

Using a large or wide grip requires *little force*.

Gripping small objects places *three times the force* on the knuckle and palm.

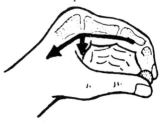

So far you have heard about the knuckles, with *subluxation* (i.e. out-of-joint), *ulnar drift* and the *Z* or *zig-zag* deformity between the wrist, knuckles and fingers. Now we shall look at the risk joints of the fingers and thumb.

The middle (or proximal) finger joint can become deformed due to joint damage and imbalance of the small muscles. This deformity is both described as, and called, a *swan-neck deformity*.

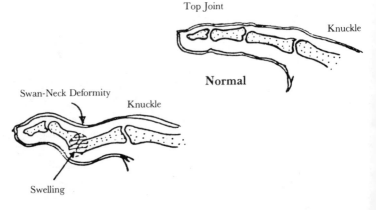

Swan-neck deformity occurs after the initial involvement of the knuckle, when a form of muscle spasm (or tightness) pulls in the direction shown by the arrows in the diagram of the swan-neck deformity.

This can then lead to the deformity shown and is known medically as *intrinsic plus*. Some activities can put undue strain on the finger and actually *encourage* it to take this abnormal position — which is why it is stressed that you should avoid certain functions.

One example of a position to be avoided is as shown below, for example, when carrying plates or trays: —

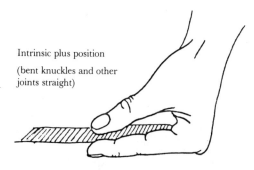

Intrinsic plus position

(bent knuckles and other joints straight)

Now let us look at the *thumb*. The thumb has three joints, all of which can be affected in the same way as the fingers.

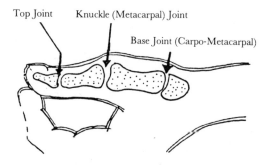

Top Joint   Knuckle (Metacarpal) Joint

Base Joint (Carpo-Metacarpal)

Starting at the base (or carpo metacarpal) joint, if this becomes inflamed, it will swell and so stretch the joint capsule. If the capsule is stretched, it allows the base joint to go out of joint (sublux). *Two* things can then happen.

If either the top joint or knuckle joint is too lax or slack, it will bend in an abnormal position, giving 2 very characteristic deformities. The following diagrams will explain this more clearly.

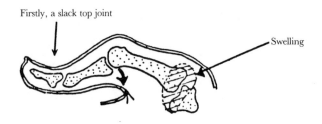

Firstly, a slack top joint

Swelling

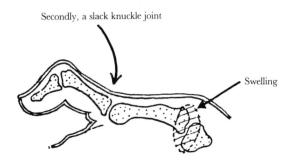

Secondly, a slack knuckle joint

Swelling

Next, the knuckle (or metacarpal) joint. When this joint is inflamed, the swelling will stretch the joint capsule and ligaments, so that it will go into the following position:—

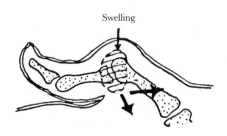

Swelling

Occasionally one of the muscle tendons which passes directly over the top of the knuckle joint may become broken (or ruptured) due to it being over-stretched by the swollen capsule. This then means that you may have difficulty in straightening your thumb.

All these joint deformities can be made worse by the way in which you use your thumb. A common example is leaning heavily on the thumb and knuckles whilst getting up from a bed or chair (see the diagram on page 43).

Now you have read this outline of hand anatomy and deformity, look through the diagrams about joint care in Chapter 7. Try and relate the situations to yourself. If necessary, read the chapter again until you are happy that you have understood it.

You will now realise that the way you use your hands can influence the way the joints behave. Joint care *cannot prevent* deformity, which is caused by the arthritis, but it *can control* it. Joint care matters and it is something that you can do for yourself. *Try it*.

Here are 5 guidelines for you:

1. Small joints cannot take great pressure (e.g. close a drawer with your rear or a foot).

2. Avoid prolonged or continuous grip — keep changing your position (e.g. little and often is better than non-stop).

3. Avoid strain on individual joints — distribute it over several joints (e.g. use both hands).

4. Avoid pressure on the knuckle joints — use larger handles if necessary.

5. Avoid handling heavy things — distribute the load (e.g. get assistance or use a trolley for suitcase or shopping).

Remember

There are very few things that you must not do. It is the way they are done that counts.

7. Guidelines for Joint Care

'For the past 8 years I have had to work out for myself how to organise my life. It would have been a great help to have had reassurance that what I was doing was right. Most people give sympathy but nothing positive. Generally I have been told *not* to do anything instead of trying to explain why doing things the normal way is damaging. I can imagine that is must be very trying having to explain a situation to 20 different patients, but where else do we go for advice? When staff have given me support and help by being positive in their outlook for me, it makes me feel part of the human race again.'

'I wish that I had received advice on the importance of joint care at the beginning and then I would not have subjected my joints to so much stress.'

This chapter explains how to take care of your joints by showing you — mostly in pictures — the right and wrong ways to perform everyday actions.

Pushing up from a chair

When pushing up from a chair, avoid using your wrists or knuckles.

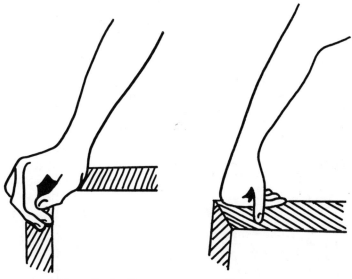

This method will
cause pain.

Extreme stress
on the knuckles.

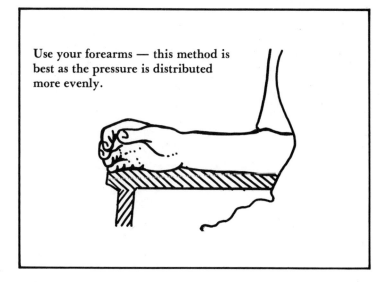

**Use your forearms — this method is
best as the pressure is distributed
more evenly.**

Getting out of a chair

When getting out of a chair *with arms*, avoid putting pressure on your knuckles or wrists and avoid straining your shoulders.

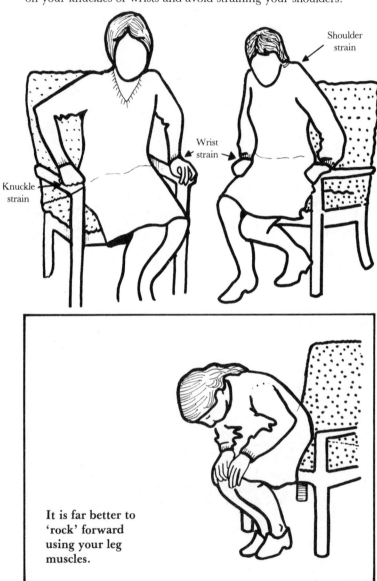

Shoulder strain

Wrist strain

Knuckle strain

It is far better to 'rock' forward using your leg muscles.

Similarly, when getting out of an *upright* chair, avoid putting pressure on your shoulders, elbows and fingers.

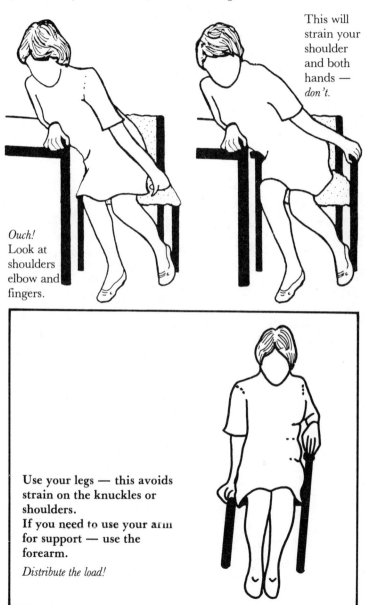

This will strain your shoulder and both hands — *don't.*

Ouch! Look at shoulders elbow and fingers.

Use your legs — this avoids strain on the knuckles or shoulders.
If you need to use your arm for support — use the forearm.
Distribute the load!

Reading a book

When reading a book avoid resting on your elbows and knuckles or elbows and wrists as these will all be strained.

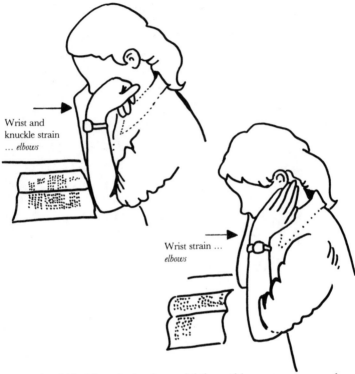

Wrist and
knuckle strain
... *elbows*

Wrist strain ...
elbows

Avoid holding the book too tightly as this can encourage ulnar drift.

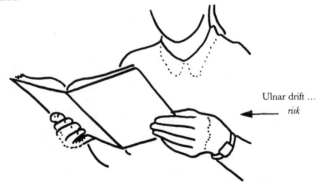

Ulnar drift ...
risk

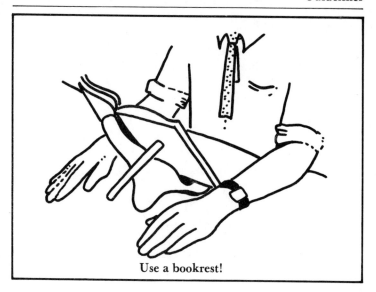

Use a bookrest!

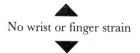

No wrist or finger strain

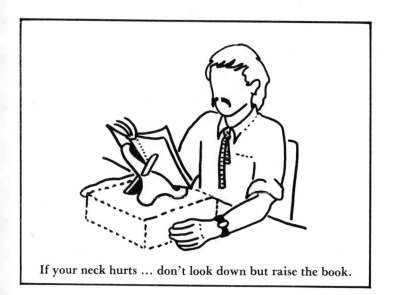

If your neck hurts ... don't look down but raise the book.

Opening a jar

Be very careful when opening a jar. If you hold the lid with your fingers and thumb and turn towards your fingers it will strain your thumb and increase the ulnar drift risk.

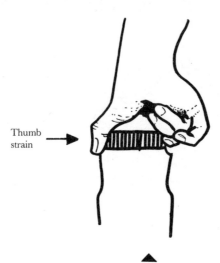

Thumb strain →

▲

Ulnar Drift — All the load is on the fingers and thumb.

▼

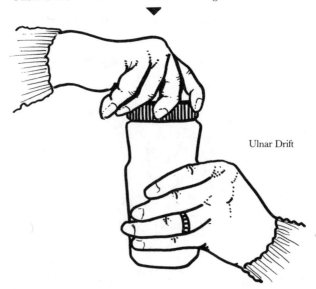

Ulnar Drift

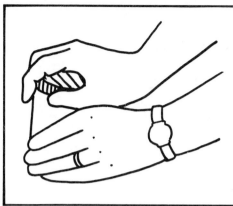

It is important to use both hands. **ALWAYS SCREW TOWARDS THE THUMB,** using the palm of the hand to increase your grip.

Rest the supporting hand on the table to discourage ulnar drift.

BETTER STILL, use an 'Unduit' V-shaped opener mounted on to a **door** *or* wall *or* underneath a shelf (this is available from hardware shops).

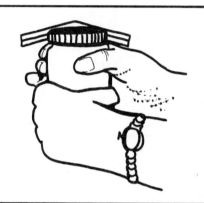

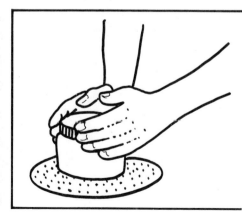

or

Use both hands on the lid and stop the jar slipping by using a non-slip mat (or damp cloth).

Carrying a bag

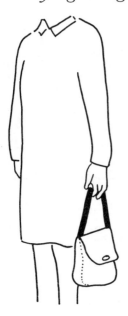

Try to avoid carrying too much weight —
handbags can be as heavy as toolbags.

Avoid carrying your bag by holding the
strap in your hand as this will cause strain on the shoulder and fingers.

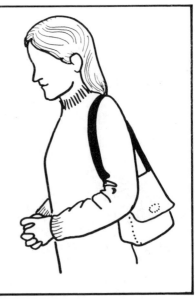

If your bag is not too heavy it is better to carry it on your shoulder.

Opening packets and tins

When opening packets try to avoid causing yourself any
unnecessary pain. *If the packet has a special opener, use it.*

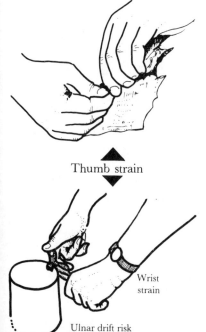

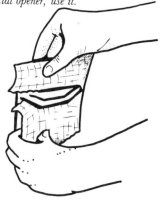

Thumb strain

When opening tins it is
best to avoid a hand
tin-opener which will
also cause you
unnecessary problems.

Wrist
strain

Ulnar drift risk

**Use a wall-mounted
style — this
distributes the
pressure more evenly.**

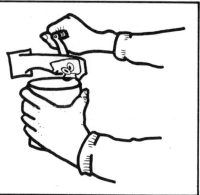

NOTE

**If your thumb is still
affected — buy a wall
tin-opener with a small
'shelf' to hold the weight
of the tin.** (Ask your
occupational therapist for
an address).

Taps

Most types of tap cause a strain on wrist, thumbs and fingers.

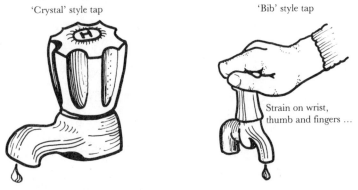

'Crystal' style tap

'Bib' style tap

Strain on wrist, thumb and fingers ...

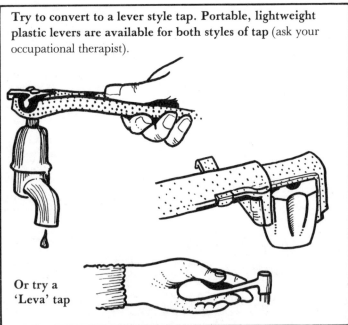

Try to convert to a lever style tap. Portable, lightweight plastic levers are available for both styles of tap (ask your occupational therapist).

Or try a 'Leva' tap

COMMON SENSE TIPS:

use a damp cloth

or

use a piece of non-slip material

Either will increase your grip on the object.

Saucepans

Try to avoid lifting saucepans with one hand.

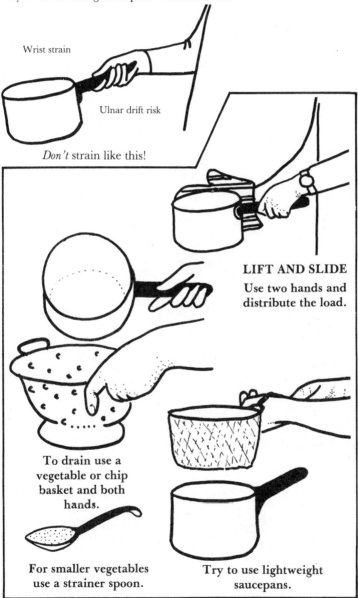

Wrist strain

Ulnar drift risk

Don't strain like this!

LIFT AND SLIDE
Use two hands and
distribute the load.

To drain use a
vegetable or chip
basket and both
hands.

For smaller vegetables
use a strainer spoon.

Try to use lightweight
saucepans.

Holding a cup

Holding a cup can cause strain on fingers and knuckles.

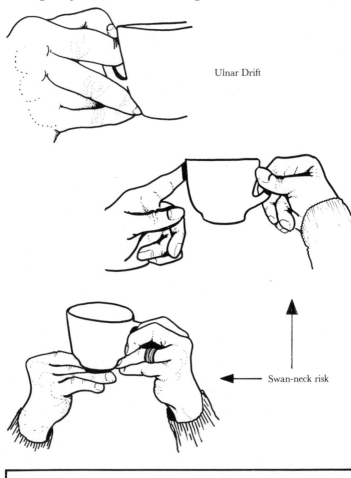

Ulnar Drift

Swan-neck risk

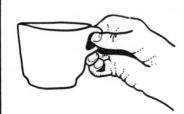

Bend the fingers at the middle joint. Use a lightweight cup or mug.

Try a larger handle (camping equipment or Melaware is ideal).

Using a teapot

Take care when using a teapot too.

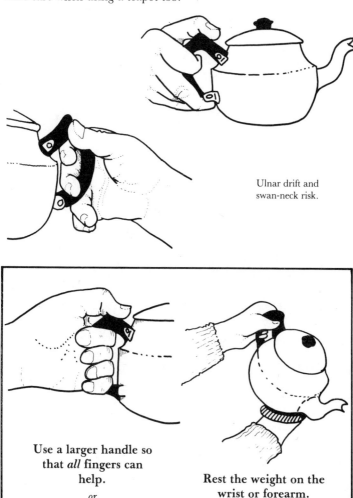

Ulnar drift and
swan-neck risk.

Use a larger handle so
that *all* fingers can
help.
or
Use both hands.

Rest the weight on the
wrist or forearm.

TIPS

A lightweight or insulated teapot will help.

Half fill if necessary.

Cutlery

Take care with your wrists and fingers when using cutlery.

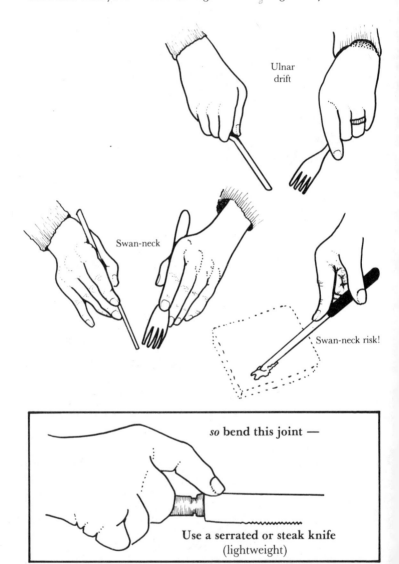

Ulnar drift

Swan-neck

Swan-neck risk!

so bend this joint —

Use a serrated or steak knife
(lightweight)

REMEMBER

If your knuckles hurt, use a larger handle.

Using the telephone

Remember the same principles when using the telephone.
Avoid strain on your thumb and wrist.

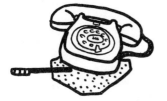

Ulnar drift risk
also
Thumb strain
Wrist strain

DON'T DIAL WITH ONE FINGER
Use a pen or pencil.
Place the telephone on a non-slip mat.

Wringing out cloths

Wringing can cause risk of
ulnar drift, as well as
straining your thumb and
wrist.

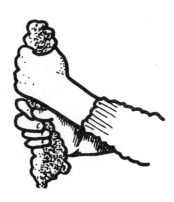

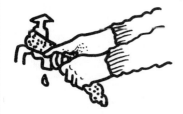

Avoid wringing out if
possible
or
**Twist the cloth
around a tap and use
both hands.**

Carrying a coat

Avoid carrying a coat like this as it puts too much strain on one finger.

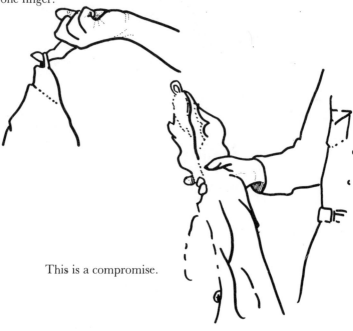

This is a compromise.

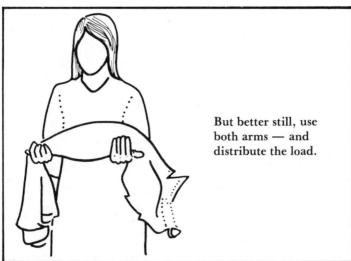

But better still, use both arms — and distribute the load.

Drawer handles

Many drawer handles can give rise to thumb and finger strain.

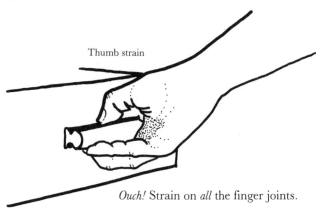

Ouch! Strain on *all* the finger joints.

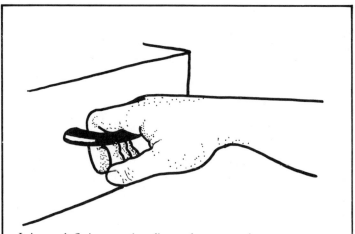

It is worth fitting new handles to drawers so that you can open them like this, distributing the strain more evenly.

REMEMBER

**Ask your occupational therapist
about joint care**

Carrying dishes

Carrying dishes can be risky.

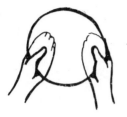

Even with both hands there is still wrist strain and ulnar drift risk.

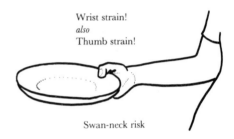

Wrist strain!
also
Thumb strain!

Swan-neck risk

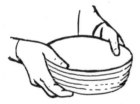

Ulnar drift risk

Wrist and finger strain

Even when you use a tray you will put strain on neck, shoulders, elbows, wrists and fingers.

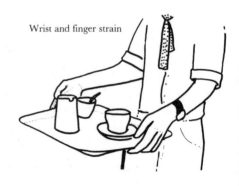

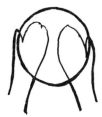

Placing both hands completely under the plate is a compromise.

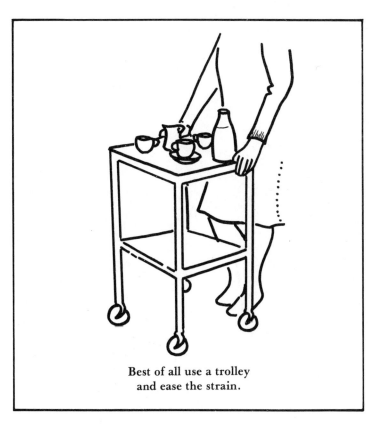

**Best of all use a trolley
and ease the strain.**

Relieving back strain

Improve your posture!

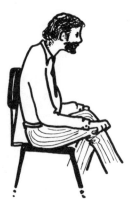

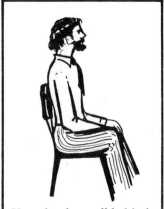

Don't slouch like this ...
Sit straight!

**Use a lumbar roll behind
your own back if possible.**

Don't bend like this ... Either
go to a hairdresser or raise
the bowl up to a better
height. If you have a shower
— stand and wash your hair.

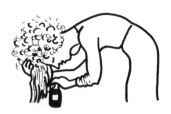

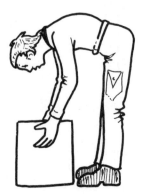

Don't lift like this!

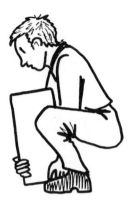

Bend your knees

and

hold the load close to your body.

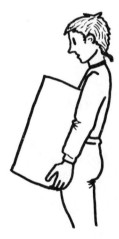

ALWAYS

Bend the knees before the back (or neck).

Rest your weight equally on both feet.

Use both sides of your body equally — to distribute the load *and* strain.

---

8. Foot Care

Pain and Discomfort

Rheumatoid arthritis often starts in the joints of the feet and most commonly the joints in the balls of the feet. In the early stages they may ache and seem stiff and swollen. Pressure on this area is usually painful — shoes don't seem to fit any more. This is because the feet have in fact *widened*, due to the swollen joints. *Do not try to force your feet into old shoes that are too tight for you.*

Later in the course of the disease, the swollen joints may force the natural cushion under the skin to move forwards, leaving the skin 'cushionless'. This lack of cushion means that the skin will have to take up to *20 times the normal pressure* — hence the discomfort when you walk or stand!

What can be done about this?

The skin can be cushioned artificially by having specially made inner soles fitted into the shoes. These inner soles are made of a special spongy material but should be fitted properly by a *State Registered Chiropodist.*

What about my shoes?

Be sensible about the type of shoes that you wear. The *more cushioning* there is in the sole of the shoe, the *more comfortable* your feet are going to be. Choose styles that give your feet good support and are easy to get on and off. Many modern shoes are now made with comfort in mind as well as fashion, so be selective!

Do not wear shoes that are going to be tight around the toes as this will encourage them to drift out of shape more quickly. In the same way, socks or stockings should not be at all restricting around the toes.

Another comfort tip is to check the height of the heel of the shoe. When standing barefoot on a flat surface, the load on the foot is equally spread between the ball of the foot and the heel. However, when wearing shoes, the higher the heel, the greater will be the pressure on the ball of the foot and the toes, as the load has been transferred forward — just like standing on tiptoe. So ladies should be sensible and try to avoid high-heeled shoes — or at least wear them as little as possible. If you must wear a heel — compromise, and don't have it too high. You *will* notice the difference.

If in doubt about choosing a good shoe — seek the advice of your chiropodist, but the following guidelines may help you:

—Shoes held on by lacing, bars or ankle straps are generally best as they stop the foot from sliding forward and so cramping the toes. Some slip-on styles are *not* good, if they are *only* kept on because of compression between the toe and the heel. Mules are similarly not recommended as you are reliant upon the toe bar to keep them in place.

—Choose a shoe with a supple and soft upper, preferably without seams that will cause pressure on the toes. This upper may or may not be leather.

—Choose soles that are well-cushioned, flexible and non-slip. Thin inflexible plastic soles will not be comfortable, neither will leather. Similarly, a thin rubber sole glued to a leather sole will not improve the comfort at all, although it will make it non-slip. For soles, synthetic materials win every time!

Remember

If you put a cushion insole into your shoe —
you will *increase* the pressure within the shoe as there
will be *less* space.

The feet, like the hands, contain a lot of small bones and joints which is why they become so inflamed and painful. Certainly, having to walk on them when they are inflamed does not help!

A Little Anatomy

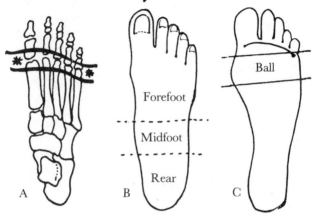

A   B   C

The metatarsal heads are the joints that are mostly affected in rheumatoid arthritis.

The feet contain many bones and joints (diagram A above) and can be divided into three areas:— the forefoot, midfoot and hind (or rear) foot (diagram B). Running from the rear foot to the ball of the foot is the longitudinal arch.

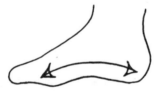

This arch has a definite function and is very important as it supports the body weight.

Muscles, tendons and *ligaments* are situated around the bones and allow for the 'springiness' and suppleness of the foot. They are responsible for the movement of the toes, as they are in the hand for the movement of the fingers.

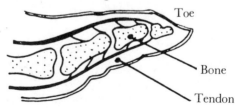

In normal circumstances, the tendons pull in a straight line (see diagram D). When, however, the joints become swollen, the tendons find themselves 'pushed' to one side — causing the muscles to pull sideways (see diagram E). This leads to a sideways deformity of the toes (diagram F) — similar to *ulnar drift* in the fingers (see Chapter 6).

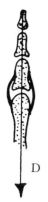 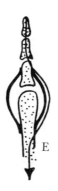 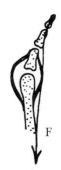

Rheumatoid arthritis also affects the joints in the *rear* of the foot, and particularly the one below the ankle joint (see diagram). The supporting structures around this joint become slack or lax, allowing the foot to 'roll over' on to its inner border:

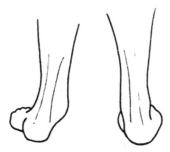

This deformity is known as *over-pronation* and gives the foot its characteristic 'flattened' appearance.

There is also another reason for this deformity. A person with painful joints in the ball of the foot (see diagram C) may turn their feet outwards to gain relief by walking on the inside edge of the foot.

Over-pronation is very bad for the mechanics of the foot — it is no longer a rigid structure with which to propel the body forwards when walking. In this weakened position the toes (and in particular, the big toe) will go 'out-of-line' very quickly. One toe may even cross over or under its neighbour, making shoes very uncomfortable.

The *knees* may also become painful due to the extra strain on them caused by the altered angle of the foot during weightbearing.

What can be done about it?

This over-pronation can be corrected to some degree — by the wearing of special splints (or orthotics) in the shoes. These rigid, functional splints are specially *made to measure* and must *only* be provided by a State Registered Chiropodist, who will measure how much correction you need. The splints look similar to arch supports but work in a different way. Arch supports will *not* correct your over-pronation.

Note

There are over 26 bones in each foot, and any one — or all — of them can be affected by arthritis! *Feet matter* — you have to walk on them — so pay them a bit more attention ....

Points to remember

Wear appropriate shoes ... supportive, plenty of room for the toes and with a good, flexible cushion sole. *Avoid* high heels.

—See a State Registered Chiropodist regularly for advice — and help to prevent problems occurring *by going early*. Look for the letters S.R.C.H. after the name — which means that the person has completed a three-year full-time course of training and is professionally approved by the National Health Service.

—When your feet are swollen and painful, *rest* them and elevate them to help the swelling to go down. When the swelling and pain settle, exercise them gently (see Chapter 5).

—Look after your skin (see Chapter 12).

—By adding padding inside the shoe you actually *increase* the pressure ... and may make things worse! A State Registered Chiropodist will advise you.

Prevention is better than cure

9. Tips on Dressing and Self-Care

Dressing

Taking care with your clothes can make a great deal of difference to your day. You may need to make some adaptations to existing clothes, and when it comes to buying new clothes there are particular things to look out for.

Buttons

If you have difficulty, check first that the button holes are not too tight, although very small buttons may need to be replaced by more manageable ones. Sometimes it can be helpful to remove very difficult buttons (for example on the collar or cuffs) and replace with Velcro. This can be done quite easily to give a normal appearance. Firstly, remove the button and sew up the button hole. Secondly, sew the button back on to the sewn-up button hole. Cut two postage-stamp-sized pieces of Velcro and sew one to where the button originally was and the other on to the opposite surface. An alternative solution to the problem of cuffs is to eliminate the difficulty of fastenings altogether by sewing a piece of elastic between the cuffs which will stretch when the hand is pushed through. Another useful tip is to use a button or rug hook on 'bad days' — simply pass the hook through the button-hole, catch the button, and pull it back through the button hole, thus completing the fastening.

Zips

Plastic zips are generally more difficult to use than metal ones — so choose your clothing carefully. If the zip has a hole in the tag, thread a piece of tape or cord through — this will improve the leverage. There is a ready-made type available which comes complete with miniature dog clip and can be bought at most large stores or haberdashers.

Ties

On days when reaching the back of the neck or holding up the arms for any length of time is difficult — *either* avoid wearing a tie that day *or* buy a ready-made elastic style.

Shoes and fastenings

You should always wear good supportive leather shoes and avoid slippers. The shoes should be wide enough to accommodate the toes comfortably and have low heels. Insoles are available from your local chemist, Scholl shop or chiropodist (see Chapter on *Foot Care*).

Modern casual shoes (e.g. Clark's) provide good foot support and often have Velcro fastenings; styles with difficult fastenings should be avoided. If laces are a problem, wear a slip-on style aided by a long-handled plastic shoehorn, available from many shoe shops or repairers. Alternatively, replace shoelaces with elastic ones. Lace the shoes and slip on using a shoehorn. If the tongue tends to fold up when the shoe is put on, punch a couple of *small* holes in it and include in the lacing up.

Outer clothes

Choose lightweight easy-care fabrics of loose-fitting styles with front fastenings. Avoid heavy woollen or sheepskin garments — warmth can easily be achieved with lightweight quilted materials or extra layers.

Cardigans are less trouble than jumpers or pullovers. A hooked, long-handled shoehorn can also help in assisting clothing over stiff shoulders.

Tights and stockings

Single-leg tights (e.g. by 'Tytex') are available, as advertised in some newspapers, from large stores such as Debenhams or by mail order. These are helpful because being separate legs, each with a waistband, they only require to be put on/off once a day. Stocking-tights are available from some shops or by mail order.

Avoid tight-fitting socks of any composition. Towelling socks usually stretch well and some women may find pop-socks helpful.

Underclothes — women

Avoid corsets or pantie girdles when wrists or hands are painful. Light-control Lycra garments can also be difficult, while loose-fitting or camisole-style knickers are easier to manage than bikini briefs.

Bras can be fastened at the front and then twisted round, or front-fastening types — if comfortable — can be worn. Alter the fastenings if necessary by substituting Velcro for hooks and eyes or join with half-an-inch of elastic and then pull the bra over the head.

Underclothes — men

Choose front-opening or boxer style shorts rather than trunks or briefs and avoid tight-fitting vests.

Trousers — men and women

Avoid tight-fitting styles and check fastenings and zips for ease of opening. Trousers with elasticated waists are particularly comfortable.

Self-Care

Here are some tips to avoid unnecessary strain on your joints.

Shaving

Lightweight disposable razors may be helpful on days when your hands or wrists are particularly painful or stiff. If you wish to use an electric or battery shaver, check different models for weight and ease of manipulation. If you prefer a wet shave, a brush and soap may be difficult on occasions, so check other methods (e.g. aerosol foam/plastic tube) for applying lather to the face.

Make-up

Use a cosmetic sponge to apply foundation as this puts less strain on your finger joints. Use make-up brushes to apply eye shadow or blusher and always select lightweight containers that are easy to open rather than tube dispensers.

Hair

Combing Adopt an easy-care hair style and use a lightweight comb or brush that goes easily through the hair (avoid metal combs and bristle brushes if you have thick hair).

Washing Either go to a hairdresser or wash your hair whilst taking a shower and ask a spouse or relative to assist you if necessary so that you can sit or stand.

Cleaning teeth

A rubber band wound round the handle of your toothbrush aids grip, but an electric toothbrush may be preferable. If your jaw is painful, use a child's brush or one with a small head (see Chapter 12).

Washing

Always sit rather than stand and use a sponge instead of a flannel because it is easier to press out excess water (using the palm of the hand or forearm). If you must use a flannel, buy one of the cheaper, thinner types as it will be lighter, hold less water and be easier to wring out.

Holding wet soap may be difficult so use liquid soap, a flannel soap-mitt, or 'soap on a rope'. Some people find soap in a foam envelope (e.g. Bronnley's) easier to grip.

Lever-style taps are best, but standard bib taps are easier to turn than the round (acrylic/metal) types. There is a simple and removable plastic lever available for all makes of bib taps, but aids for the round-headed styles are more cumbersome. A wet cloth or piece of non-slip material such as Dycem will improve your grip (see Chapter 7).

A shower is less effort than a bath and there are now inexpensive shower/tap adaptations available on the market which do away with the necessity of fitting a complete shower unit.

Safety

Always have a non-slip surface on the bottom of the bath or shower. If you use a bath mat, choose one with as many suckers as possible, to maximise grip. Alternatively there are many attractive forms of self-adhesive strips available from large stores. If your bath has no handle, then gain extra grip by placing a wet flannel on the side of the bath as you climb in and out.

For those with painful knees, a bath board or stool may help — ask your occupational therapist for advice on the modern lightweight styles that are now available.

For those with painful elbows or shoulders, washing the neck, back, legs or feet can be a problem. Larger branches of Boots stock a useful length of flannelling with plastic hoops at both ends which can help reduce this difficulty.

Drying

Make sure your bathroom is warm, wear a towelling robe and pat yourself dry or use a lightweight towel.

WC

On your 'off' days always wear suitable clothing that requires minimum manipulation. If your knees are very painful and you find it difficult to get down to the WC seat, don't be ashamed to borrow or hire a temporary plastic/polythene seat raise. This will save you a lot of discomfort and effort but it can be removed when not required either by yourself or your family. Being light-weight and hygienic, it can easily be stored in a cupboard if its presence embarrasses you. Remember it is far better not to struggle, so as to save stress on your joints at a time when they require a little care. You can always return the aid — it is not a fixture!

10. General Hints

Remembering that you are always aiming to avoid unnecessary strain on your joints, this chapter gives some general hints that may help.

Scissors

Always use lightweight, efficient scissors, with reasonable-sized handles, or ask somebody else to help you.

There are some scissors available called 'Stirex' scissors (see below).

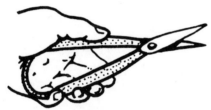

The piece of plastic which connects the blades acts as a spring, therefore only one action is required (i.e. closing the blades); they will then open themselves.

Writing

Find a pen that you can use easily, without needing much pressure (for example a felt-tipped pen). A rubber band around the pen will not only prevent it from slipping but also mean that you will not have to grip the pen so tightly.

Door handles (household)

Lever types are the most successful as the forearm can be used when the hand or wrist is painful.

Latches can be a problem if the door is not properly lined up, or the thumb is painful.

Round handles can also be a problem where there may be weakness or painful finger joints. A piece of non-slip material (Dycem) may give you more grip on the handle although it won't solve the problem.

**Ensure that all doors are properly maintained
— a stiff handle could be remedied by oiling!**

Keys

The problem with most keys is lack of leverage, therefore add some by any one of the following methods:

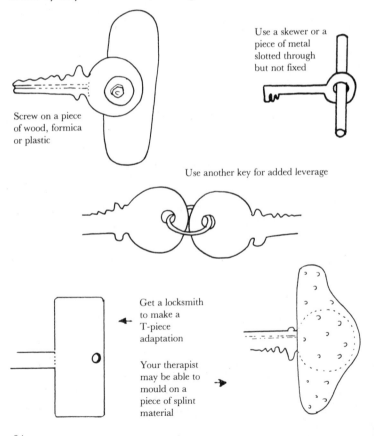

Screw on a piece of wood, formica or plastic

Use a skewer or a piece of metal slotted through but not fixed

Use another key for added leverage

Get a locksmith to make a T-piece adaptation

Your therapist may be able to mould on a piece of splint material

Handling money

Pushing hands in pockets or into purses can be difficult when finger joints are either swollen or painful. A gent's purse (available from large stores or Boots) may be useful here:—

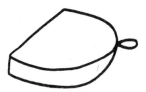 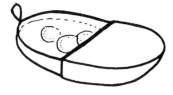

When open this purse provides a flat 'shelf' to sort coins and a 'lip' to enable coins to be picked up more easily. However, if choosing one, select one in a softer, thinner leather (usually the cheapest) as these are the easiest to open. Avoid styles that include a catch or press fastening and note that some styles also have a separate pocket for notes, which can be useful.

Public transport

There are no short cuts to using public transport — but do take heed of the following tips:—

Never try to board a bus or train at the last minute — stiff joints may make you less nimble than you thought!

Similarly — never leave a bus or train before it has completely stopped and you are ready, and if travelling on buses, be careful if your fingers are more stiff than normal — lest they 'hook' around the pole on the bus platform.

On main line trains, it may be necessary, in sufficient time before the destination, to ask somebody to help you to open the door — it may save you from unnecessary pain!

Cars

Keys

If the lock is stiff — get it checked. If the key is too small — investigate means of adding leverage (see section on keys), taking into consideration the amount of space available to turn the key.

Door handles

Keep them well-maintained to prevent stiffness. If necessary, here is a portable/temporary way of increasing leverage:—

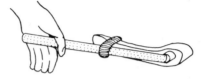

Hand brake

If you find this difficult — check with your local garage as some will adapt it for you.

General

Automatic cars are obviously less of a problem than cars with a manual gear change. However, some types of gear change may be more suitable for you than others. You may find it beneficial to wear wrist supports whilst driving — see your therapist.

11. Why Splint?

As soon as a joint becomes swollen, it is at risk, and so splints are an excellent way of resting the joint to help the swelling go down.

You do not need to have deformities to have splints. In fact, it is better to have splints just as *soon as your joints become swollen, hot and painful.*

Some joints are easier to splint than others, and the most commonly splinted ones are the hands (including fingers), wrists, elbows, neck, knees and feet. *That does not mean that all your joints will be splinted at the same time!* You may only need a splint for your wrist or fingers — so don't imagine being enclosed in a suit or armour ....

Splints have several different functions:

To protect or support ... one painful joint. (For example, the wrist whilst the rest of the limb is used.)

To rest ... one or more joints that are inflamed (for example, whilst you are in bed).

To prevent ... joints going 'out-of-line', especially whilst they are affected by the swelling.

To keep still ... it may be necessary to stop a joint from moving in order to help the inflammation go down.

But splinting will be under supervision so that you don't get too stiff!

'I am 32 years old and have had RA for 9 years. I wish that I had known earlier just how importants splints were in helping to prevent deformity and as a resting aid. I feel that if better, neater, more comfortable splints had been given to me earlier, I would now be so bad now as I might actually have worn them. As it was, the huge clumsy, pink things I was given were so off-putting, both to me and my husband (and not very sexy!) that I didn't wear them.'

Splints can be divided up into day and night splints. The most common ones are the paddle splint, wrist support and collar.

Firstly, the *paddle splint*. This is a complete resting splint for the wrist, hand and fingers. It can be worn either at night or when resting during the day.

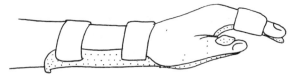

Note: The straps or design may vary a little.

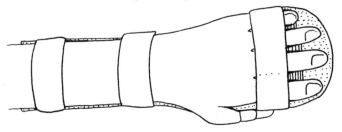

The *wrist splint* is also known as the wrist resting splint, wrist working splint or wrist gauntlet!

Its function is to support and keep the wrist still, whilst enabling you to use your fingers. This helps greatly in reducing wrist pain.

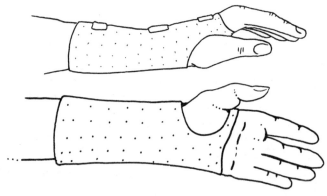

Sometimes these splints are made from an elastic material with a strengthener along the front of the wrist into the palm. However, like all mass-made items, this type may not fit you —

and an *exact* fit is crucial if the splint is to be comfortable. Therefore, your therapist may have to make you a special one, to your own requirements, but it will *not* be in elastic.

A *collar* is sometimes recommended if your neck is very painful. There are two types, for day or night wear. A night collar is far less rigid than a day one — to enable you to sleep in it. A collar for day use should be a good fit, so that you *cannot* move your head in any direction! If you can move your head, then the joints in your neck will not get any rest. *But*, just because the collar has to be rigid does not mean that it must be bulky and unsightly. Your therapist will show you what can be done.

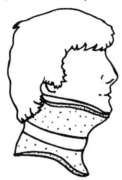

There are many different types of splints, but this should serve as an introduction for you.

Materials

Modern materials are lightweight, more attractive and fairly quick and easy to work with. A form of plastic that can be made soft in hot water is very popular, as it can be moulded directly *on you* with the minimum of pressure — *and* when no hotter than a bowl of washing-up water! It can also be perforated.

Sometimes plastic mesh or a foam-like material may be used. The foam-like material has to be cooked in an oven and so takes a little longer to make. Ask your therapist to show you what will be used. The choice of material — and even design — will depend upon your needs.

If you have an allergy to man-made materials or sticking plaster, or even if you are prone to heat-rash, *do mention it before the splint is started.*

Plaster of Paris is still used, but is not so popular because of its bulk and weight.

Don't forget — splints can be perforated, so ask for it to be done if you feel they are going to be too hot to wear.

The design of the splint will obviously depend upon its purpose — but your therapist will take special care to ensure that it is neither too heavy, awkward nor ugly. *Nobody* wants to wear anything too unsightly or cumbersome!

Don't panic: Your therapist will treat you gently — tell them *where* it hurts!

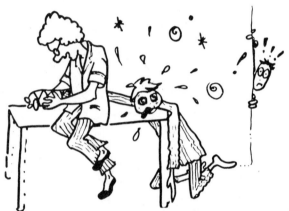

There! That was easy wasn't it?

Modern materials are much easier to use. Your therapist will tell you how hot the material is *before* it is moulded to you ... so don't panic!

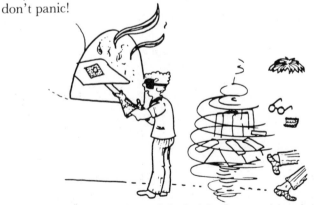

Now this is *not* as hot as it looks Mr. Jones ... just relax.

Points to note

Wear the splint when you are advised to. If you are not told — or don't understand — *ask again*, get the therapist to write it down. *Remember — it is their job!*

If the splint is not comfortable, mention it at once. If at home, take the splint off, *then* contact the therapist for another appointment. *Never* continue to wear it if it hurts — any more than you would wear the wrong sized shoes.

Your therapist will need to see you at least once after making the splint — to check its fit. If alterations are necessary, several visits will be planned.

Do allow enough time if a splint has to be specially made for you, although alterations take less time. Again, ask your therapist to advise you but as a general guideline — allow one hour per splint (to include strapping) ... some may be a lot quicker than this.

Splints are often called *orthoses* by the medical profession. This is a more modern term, but as far as you are concerned — it is the same thing.

Never, never wear anybody else's splint. To do its job properly, the splint must have been made to fit you — and you only!

Splinting cannot cure ... but it can help

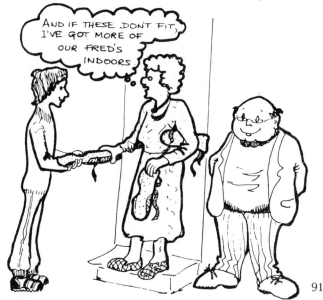

12. Skin and Body Care

When you are experiencing a 'flare-up' of your rheumatic disease it is important that you rest as much as possible. During that period it is advisable that you take a little more care of your *skin* and pressure points to avoid any damage.

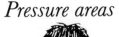

Pressure areas

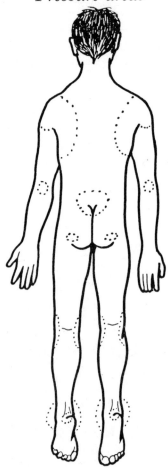

Bathing

Your joints may feel much more relaxed after a bath or shower using either tepid or hot water. Find out which time of the day a bath is most beneficial to your aching joints, morning or evening.

An evening bath may relax your joints and enable you to have a good night's sleep. A morning bath may help to reduce stiffness in your joints.

If you find your skin is becoming dry, use a bath oil; this will help to nourish your skin. Be careful to use a bath oil that does not make your bath slippery. Always have a non-slip bath mat at the bottom of your bath.

If you have difficulty getting in and out of your bath, use a bath seat; this will allow you to get in and out much more easily.

Ask your occupational therapist where you can get one, and which model would be most suitable for your needs.

Ensure that you dry your skin very thoroughly and do not leave any damp areas. If you find this hard work, wrap yourself into a bathrobe or towel and pat yourself dry. Do not rub your skin, this can cause minor damage.

Check your body daily for abrasions especially if you wear splints from time to time.

Use a light dusting of your favourite talcum powder when finished.

If you have particular problems with your shoulders or have a severe flare-up, you may find a longer-lasting deodorant such as 'Odaban' useful.

Make-up

Use your favourite make-up in order to look your best. It will cheer you up.

If you find that some heavily perfumed brands don't suit you so well, switch to a different make-up. Always use light-weight applications. Look in the chapter *Tips on Dressing and Self-Care* for useful tips and hints.

Rest

When your joints are painful and you rest for periods during the day, make sure that you are in a comfortable sitting position, so that there is no pressure on your painful joints.

Your back should be straight, your neck supported, shoulders and elbows should be in a comfortable resting position, and your feet should be up on a stool.

If you are resting in bed, a light-weight continental quilt relieves the weight from your knees, ankles and feet. A stool at the bottom of your bed will help to lift heavy bed clothing and support your feet.

Beware though that you don't hit your legs and feet on anything hard which could produce a skin breakage.

If your elbows get sore from frequently changing your position, protect them with light elbow pads made from sheepskin or other soft material. The same applies to your heels. Ask your therapist or nurse for advice.

If you develop small nodules on your elbows, hands, knees or feet, be sure to keep them free from pressure. Consult your doctor if they become tender and painful.

Splints

You may have been given resting splints to wear in order to immobilise your affected joint or joints for a period.

If they are too tight and feel uncomfortable take them back to your therapist to have them altered. Never allow your skin to become red and tender from ill-fitting splints.

The same applies to your *working* splints or your collar.

Never wear uncomfortable or ill-fitting shoes. Blisters can develop into sores and can take a long time to heal.

If a sore develops, ensure that you keep it clean. Use a little cream, such as Savlon, and cover with a pad and bandage.

Avoid using plaster on your skin
Avoid any further pressure
Do take special care

Exercises

You will have been advised to do your exercises regularly to keep your joints mobile. This may make you perspire more. It is important to prevent any rashes developing because of perspiration. Check your skin regularly, wash and dry well after your exercises.

Feet

See your chiropodist at regular intervals to keep your feet well looked after. If you are unable to have regular baths, soak your feet in warm water. If the skin becomes dry, use moisturising, non-perfumed cream for your feet. *The best and mildest ones are still the various baby creams and lotions.* (See also chapter on *Foot Care.*)

Eyes

You may experience a dry and gritty feeling in your eyes from time to time. Your eyes may become sore and look red; this could be due to dryness of the eyes. The problem can easily be rectified. See your doctor; he will usually give you eye-drops to keep your eyes moist. Ask the nurse at the surgery to teach you how to use them.

Teeth

Looking after teeth can be a problem for many people but particularly if you have very painful or stiff shoulders, elbows, wrists, hands or jaws. Teeth care should not be overlooked. Poor oral hygiene leads to gum infections and tooth decay. *These can then trigger 'flare-ups' of your arthritis.*

Another important factor in dental decay is dry mouth, caused by lack of saliva. If you have this problem, see your doctor or dentist and ask for advice.

Toothbrushes

A toothbrush normally has a rather short, thin handle. If it becomes difficult to manage due to stiffness or pain, the handle can be easily modified:

Wind a rubber band around the handle to provide more grip.

Enlarge the handle with foam (see fig. A).

Buy a toothbrush with a thicker handle — travelling models are ideal (see fig. B).

Buy a preformed enlarged foam handle (such as 'plastazote') from large chemist shops (see fig. C).

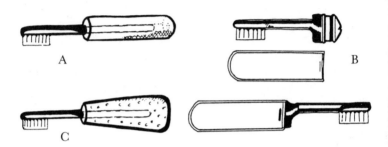

Take care of your body

With a little extra care you can keep your skin smooth and free from pressure and sores.

13. Coping with a Young Family: a personal experience

I developed rheumatoid when my youngest son was exactly one year old. Although I am unable to make any practical suggestions for coping with totally helpless infants, the following discoveries and experiences might be useful to people in a similar situation.

Help is the first essential. It is very tiring caring for young children even when you have your full health and strength. It becomes almost impossible when you have a disease which drains your energy even more. Help comes in many shapes and forms and everyone can manage to make use of some of the simpler forms even if you are unable to afford professional help. Do not forget, however, that your local health visitor is often able to supply a temporary helper at small cost if you are really stuck. I employed all the methods described in Chapter 3.

It is never to early to start training the baby. At a very early age my little one would collect his nappy and changing things, clean socks etc. and could load all the dirty clothes into the washing machine in a twinkling of an eye. He is growing up to be very useful at those jobs around knee level! It is a good thing to take advantage (only not too much of course!) of this early eagerness to help. It soon passes.

Once you have made day-to-day life easier for yourself, it's on to caring for the baby.

Caring for the Baby

Lifting

This, of course, is one of the worst problems. Babies need to be lifted and cuddled but this puts great strain on your joints.

Cuddling lying down is very good. You can both be supported by the bed and get really close to each other without too much damage being inflicted on your weary joints. Similarly, if you are sitting down and there is someone else present, ask them to lift the baby on to your lap to save the strain of lifting.

For a child that can stand I devised a method of lifting which puts the weight on to the forearm instead of on to the shoulders and hands. Stand behind the child and put your arm between his legs. Put your other arm around his waist and draw him back so he is sitting on your forearm. Draw him closer to your body as you lift so that your arms and body take the weight with the encircling arm just steadying him and stopping him from falling. After a while the child becomes used to this method and helps. My little one would shout from his cot and stand with arms held up in the usual way. If it was I and not his father who appeared he would simply turn round ready to be lifted from behind. By the time the child is 2 you can probably get away with a fireman's lift to transport him downstairs etc. if he will suffer this. Another tip is to lift from a higher surface. I found it very difficult to lift from floor level but once he was able to scramble up on to a chair and stand up it all became much easier. Also if we wanted to go downstairs, I would stand him on the top step and go down a few steps myself first before lifting. I cannot however solve the problem of what to do when you want to move him. I fear patience and waiting for him to get bored and get up again is the only answer. If he wants to sit up I offer a forearm and he clasps it.

Washing and dressing

Right from the start I insisted on the baby lying down for washing. Unless you are able to kneel easily, I do not recommend bathing. Bath time was a special treat supervised by father and as such was not an everyday occupation. Overall washing is quite sufficient. If you are able to get on the floor, washing, changing and dressing is probably easiest on the bathroom floor. I was not able to do this and so have always used a waterproof changing mat on a higher surface. For me the ideal height is on top of my bed. I tried using the cot for a while to stop him rolling about, but it was a little too confined and as I never left him alone on the bed this proved to be the best place.

Inability to wring out flannels etc. proved a problem and in the end I found the least messy way was as follows. Place a towel under the baby on the waterproof mat to absorb any excess water and prevent it seeping up under the baby's back. Have two small bowls of lukewarm water on a chair, table or other raised surface beside you (not on the bed where the baby can knock it over). I used small round litre ice-cream tubs as they were ideal size and weight: larger containers became hard to carry when full of water. As I also used disposable nappies in large economy packs I used the boxes as my table. If you have good grip and control of your fingers cotton-wool is probably preferable to a flannel but I found this too fiddly and finally settled for baby sponges which can be 'wrung' by simply pressing flat. I used one colour for face and one for bottom, utilising my two bowls. I continued to use this method until my son was well able to stand at the sink and help himself in washing.

Dressing the baby is even more difficult than dressing yourself because everything is so much smaller. Choose the simplest clothes with a minimum of fastenings and especially no small fiddly buttons. (N.B. Choose clothes in easy care, non-iron material where possible.) Wide or envelope necks are ideal and you can replace hooks and eyes or poppers with Velcro if you can't manage them. My greatest discovery here was Velcro trainers which proved to be a boon for mum and baby alike. We both wear them now and he can easily manage fastening them for himself. Buy snowsuits or outer clothes in large sizes to make pulling them on easier and if you are visiting enlist the hostess' aid to dress him up before going home.

For fastening conventional shoes and sandals or putting on socks I found it a useful idea to sit him on the stairs just a couple of steps up so that I could reach him easily.

Nappies

Unless you are dexterous with pins and able to push them through several layers of terry nappies I would forget all about such nappies. I still had a supply of terries from my previous baby but decided to throw economy to the winds because of the saving in energy with disposables. I did still have some difficulty unpicking the sealing tags but 'Pampers' have two tags on top of each other (for resealing nappies which turn out to be dry) and I usually managed to unpick one or both of these. Failing that, you can cut them off! The overwhelming advantage, of course, is not having to launder them, saving energy in washing, lifting and pegging out washing. Buy them in bulk and try to think of the cost of electricity and washing powder if you were using terries.

I found nappy-changing the hardest thing — very time-consuming and more and more difficult as the baby grew and became unco-operative. If you can rope anyone in to do it for you at any time, take advantage of it. If you are not able to lift the baby's legs to slip the nappy underneath, employ the bed-bath method and roll. Position the nappy close to one side of the baby, roll him, by pushing his back and bottom gently, on to his side and edge the nappy right up to the small of his back. The roll him back on to it. Roll him the other way and pull the nappy further. It takes patience and practice but you can soon become quite deft at it. We decided not to pot too early to save all the struggle with continual dressing and undressing.

Feeding

I tried to include the toddler into the family meals timetable as soon as possible, both to save energy on cooking extra meals and to make sure I had assistance at most meals.

I never satisfactorily solved the problem of a comfortable height for the baby's chair when I was on my own with him. A high chair is wonderful for the actual feeding, but very difficult to get the baby in and out of, especially if you have a fixed table top so that the baby has to be lifted high and slotted in. It is easier when the child can stand and climb a bit. Mine would scramble on to a chair to be lifted the rest of the way to his high chair. To come out I would seize him under the arms from behind and help him to stand and then fireman's lift him from there. A low chair may be better but I personally found it very difficult to get down low enough to feed him or was unable to get up again. While the baby is young enough, sitting propped up in the pram, amply swathed in protective clothing, is undoubtedly the easiest.

Spurn most of the available feeding/training cups. They are impossible to take the lid off without much strain on the joints.

Until you can persuade him to use an ordinary cup, try the one manufactured by Maws, which is a threaded screw top and very easy unless you screw it up with more force than you probably possess.

Decant large bottles of squash etc. into smaller ones. (If you buy giant economy washing powder packs, do the same with those.)

Going out

When I first asked the experts if there were any ideas for managing a pushchair and taking the baby out, I was told I would have to stay at home. This is not only not true, it is very bad for both mother and baby never to be able to go out alone together. The first thing to remember is that pushing a chair and even walking with a toddler is quite tiring, and when I intend to go out, I plan to do very little else of high-energy level during the rest of the day. Forget all about coachbuilt heavy pushchairs and prams and invest in the lightweight buggy-style with high handles. I found the Maclaren's middle-priced buggy the best. I do not advise having the style with swivel wheels. For me, it was rather like driving a supermarket trolley with a will of its own and I found it utterly impossible to control.

The next problem was harnessing the baby. The buggy comes with a very simple round-the-waist and between-the-legs strap which is easy to do up but I was concerned about the safety of this. I used a Mothercare safety harness to which a rein could be attached and used it for the pushchair, highchair and for walking. However, these have to be attached to two small anchor points in the seat of the chair. They are awkward to get at and fitted with dog-lead clips which are too stiff for a rheumatoid patient to operate. We solved this problem by making a single purchase which gave me total freedom. Go to a shop selling climbing or sailing gear and buy some carabina clips in a fairly modest size. These are used for clipping ropes together. They remain firmly closed in use but are opened easily by simply pressing down lightly on one bar. These we attached to the dog-lead clips and they remain permanently in position on the harness, to be clipped to the anchor points on anything I need or simply to attach the walking reins.

The next thing was the question of the handles. The buggy is a very good height for an average-sized adult and there is no need to crouch over it. However, I found the handles rather painful to grasp so we covered these with pieces of rubber/polystyrene tubing which fit neatly over the handles, giving a thicker gripping surface and a cushioned edge. Thus equipped, straightforward walking is easy.

If you have difficulty dragging the chair round to turn the corner, simply lean down hard with your forearms to start the swing, and if necessary hook the handles over your elbows to lift and turn it. This is also the best method to go up kerbs and steps. Stop at the step. Lean down hard on the handles with your arms so that the front wheels come up and rest on the kerb. Complete the movement by hooking the handles over the inner elbows and push the back of the chair on to the step. With a little practice this can be done quickly and neatly.

If the child is walking, do use the reins. They are not popular nowadays but if you train your children from the beginning they will accept them and you feel much more secure knowing you can grab them quickly or hang on to them if they decide to make a run for it. Better still, if you have a lot of shopping to do take someone else with you if it is possible. At one time I even used the reins indoors to be able to get a better grip on an erring toddler.

Resting

When the baby is still quite small and having several naps a day, let him sleep downstairs in a carrycot, pram or even a second cot, to save several unnecessary trips up and downstairs. Accustom him early to sleeping in 'the thick of things' and he will take no notice of the hoovering and other signs of daily life. Mine conceived a great liking for the central heating boiler and liked to sleep near it so that the noise lulled him off to sleep.

Make at least one period of the day a time for joint resting. It is really worth ignoring the chores and having a set time every day to put your feet up. We made it a rule even when my little one grew past much sleep that he and I went to lie on our beds for half to one hour every day and I found this invaluable for recharging batteries before the school age ones arrived home. We did this immediately after lunch.

Now there are no day-time rests, but I try to ensure that we put our feet up on the sofa for a while after lunch and read a book together or watch children's lunchtime programme. I certainly notice the days we don't.

Social life

This I found the hardest to cope with. Neither of us had any social life in the early days but I gradually cultivated one or two sensible friends who would bring their children round to play occasionally. They would never outstay their welcome, would help providing drinks, trips to the loo, referee fights etc. so that I wasn't continually up and down like a yo-yo, and these visits provided a pleasant interlude for both of us. Discourage visitors who watch you make the coffee, leave their cups on the floor, allow their children to ransack the house and finally leave just when supper is due and you are totally exhausted. You cannot afford to be so long-suffering as you once were!

After a while we began to pay short visits to other people, which made a pleasant change. I still find it difficult to cope with vast hordes and for this reason we did not persevere long with mums and toddlers although certainly my son enjoyed the rough and tumble. Instead we joined the National Childbirth Trust which has branches in most areas and runs good supportive services, social events and regular coffee mornings. This introduced my son into groups of children which were not too overpowering in number for either of us.

I think it is important to strike the balance between contact with other children and exhausting yourself. It has to be said, too, that the more they mix with others the more boisterous they become at home, so take it slowly and only as you are able to cope with more things. If you have a friend willing to take your child to the park sometimes you are very fortunate. We have not had this chance very often and as we have only a small garden working off excess energy is not easy. I decided to sacrifice the carpets etc. and allow a trike indoors. If you have the room this helps.

Don't forget your own social life. I usually found when my son was very small that I had no energy to go out in the evenings either alone or with my husband nor did I feel like giving dinner parties or entertaining. I tended to look for daytime activities that I could do with my son: we did N.C.T. (as above). Look out for groups at the local church where the babies are looked after and the mums study, talk or have services, babysitting coffee mornings etc. I was able to find a rehabilitation swimming session at the local sports centre for people with handicaps to swim in hot water with a creche available.

Later I progressed to entertaining friends to coffee and biscuits, which need not be too taxing, at weekends, and I have found that as my condition improves and the children get older we are getting more and more back to a normal social life.

14. Personal Relationships

People with rheumatoid arthritis often seek medical help, but rarely for worries or physical problems concerning the more intimate aspects of relationships with their partner.

This section aims at attacking the 'taboo' on the subject, to encourage you to discuss your anxieties with your partner, to seek help together, and to write for helpful publications (addresses to be found at the end of this chapter).

Communication

This is *vital*. Discuss your feelings and problems with your partner. Seek to find solutions in a loving and caring atmosphere; don't let problems get out of proportion. It may be that you choose to seek further counselling (preferably together) from either your doctor, marriage guidance counsellor, family planning organisation or SPOD (Sexual and Personal Relationships of the Disabled — address to be found at the end of this chapter).

Remember

Do discuss your feelings with your partner and/or family

Planning

Careful planning applies to all aspects of life for the arthritic — not least sex. Think carefully about organising your work to save and conserve energy. Use labour-saving gadgets or equipment wherever possible. Give yourself ample opportunity to rest e.g. by using nursery schools for small children, and to off-load work e.g. home help schemes. PLAN your work *and* leisure time and be realistic about how much you can do at a time. Careful planning will help you not to become over-tired, and leave you energy to enjoy sex. There may be certain times of the day when mobility, energy and comfort are at their highest — so if at all possible, make use of this period for sexual activity.

Self-care and interest

An important aspect of sex is feeling sexually attractive and so it is important to maintain your interest in personal care and grooming. Make sure that clothes can be easily cared for e.g. non-crease, non-iron, and where it may be difficult to look after hair, a weekly visit either to or from a hairdresser may help.

Personal care may become difficult at some stages due to pain, stiffness or flare-up. Help and advice is always available to you from your occupational therapist and through your doctor.

It is often difficult to feel attractive when depressed, anxious or just plain feeling unwell. *Everybody*, not just the arthritic, needs reassurance that they are still attractive to their partner and needed. A little pampering goes a long way towards increasing feelings of well-being — so *tell your partner how you feel* — don't burden yourself with unnecessary problems. Don't misinterpret your partner's or family's apparent lack of physical contact or interest as neglect. It is very easy for them to feel that they are undermining your independence if too enthusiastic, often to the extreme of appearing uninterested. Similarly a spouse may be so afraid of hurting painful joints that physical contact, whether casual or intimate, is avoided altogether.

You need to reassure your spouse that they can touch you without hurting you — and that gentle cuddling and caressing is more likely to make you feel better than worse.

Remember

Do discuss your feelings with your partner
and/or family

General health

Be sure to maintain general mobility and range of movement in all joints, by a regular exercise programme (see appropriate section) but *don't overdo it.*

Prior to lovemaking, hot or cold packs may ease painful joints or muscles. Similarly a hot or cold bath (or shower) may relieve pain and tension. Do make sure that your bedroom is at a comfortable temperature so that you and your partner are able to relax.

Medication

The taking of pain-killers prior to lovemaking can reduce discomfort, *but discuss any medication with your doctor.*

Some types of medication may affect your sexual activity, for example treatment for insomnia or depression may lower your sexual desire. If you have *any* doubts at all consult your doctor.

Positioning and methods

Pain and joint stiffness may make lovemaking more difficult due to problems in the hip joints of the woman or the knee and elbow joints in the man. This pain may also reduce interest in sex, which is a pity as it is a very important part of a healthy relationship. There are many positions which may be more comfortable — although intercourse is not always necessary for mutual pleasure. Many couples find great pleasure in touching and caressing without going on to have intercourse. In fact some arthritis sufferers have commented on how much more they have discovered about each other and how to give one another pleasure since intercourse has become more difficult. So, for some people, lovemaking can become more enjoyable than before.

Several information sheets and books are available on the topic (see the list at the end of this chapter) and one in particular gives specific suggestions as to how to overcome mechanical problems caused by stiff or painful joints. However, leaflets or books are not always as reassuring as discussion of worries or problems — with both your partner and a trained counsellor. SPOD have counsellors in some areas, who are always willing to listen and give advice — but if you feel that you would prefer somebody local then check with them as to who is trained and available near to you. You could also check with your local Family Planning Association or Marriage Guidance Council.

107

Try not to be embarrassed as mechanical problems with lovemaking can put unnecessary stress on a marriage at a time when, because you feel unwell, you may also be short-tempered with your 'other-half'!

In some instances cushions (or even splints) may be needed to support painful joints. They should not be avoided if they relieve pain, which may kill desire as effectively as tiredness and tension.

Guilty or Not Guilty?

Guilt is a huge barrier, all too often built up within close families. There is the guilt following angry outbursts at someone who 'was only trying to help', and the guilt of self-pity. However there is also the guilt of the carer, for expressing anger at someone who is continually tired or cross due to pain, or for their partner (or child) being affected whilst they are fit and healthy.

Guilt barriers need demolishing before they become permanent fixtures. Understanding and a little 'give and take' is needed on all sides. The carer needs a chance to let off steam as much as the sufferer! Support groups or counsellors can help a great deal — USE THEM.

Addresses and Helpful Literature

SPOD (Sexual and Personal Relationships for Disabled People), 286 Camden Road, London N7 0BJ. Tel: 01-607 8851/2. Offers a comprehensive advisory, counselling and information service, which is available to everybody.

Leaflet 6 *Sex and Arthritis*

Leaflet 7 *Positions for sex for people suffering from arthritis.*

ARC (Arthritis and Rheumatism Council), Faraday House, 8 Charing Cross Road, London WC2. ARC have local branches nationwide; they are concerned with fund raising and arthritis research.

Arthritis Care, 6 Grosvenor Crescent, London SW1 7ER. Tel: 01-235 0902/5. Arthritis Care have local branches nationwide; they are concerned with arthritis welfare and have a very active *35 Group* (address as above) for education and support for the younger arthritic.

Citizens Advice Bureau. See your local Yellow Pages.

Marriage Guidance Council. See your local Yellow Pages.

Entitled to Love by Dr Wendy Greengross. A book about disability and sex.

Marriage, Sex and Arthritis. Free booklet produced by the Arthritis and Rheumatism Council (ARC).

Advice and Equipment for Disabled People

DLF (Disabled Living Foundation), 380-384 Harrow Road, London W9 2HU. Tel: 01-289 6111.

An advisory exhibition centre run by experienced personnel and used by consumers and professionals.

The following are suppliers of Aids and Equipment for disabled people. Individual items may be obtained by mail order although prices may vary according to the quantity ordered. Details available on request.

Homecraft Supplies Ltd., 27 Trinity Road, London SW17 7SF. Tel: 01-672 7070/1789.

Nottingham Medical Aids Ltd., 17 Ludlow Hill Road, Melton Road, West Bridgford, Nottingham, NG2 6HD. Tel: 0602-234251.

Special Shops. Over the past few years several shops (such as larger branches of Boots the Chemist) have either started to sell equipment in addition to other stock or have started to specialise in aids alone. You can find your local stockist by checking in Yellow Pages (under *Disabled — Vehicles and Equipment*). However, it is far better — unless replacing existing equipment — to get advice before buying aids which could later prove to be an expensive mistake. TRY BEFORE YOU BUY! Get yourself referred either to a physiotherapist (for walking and mobility problems) or an occupational therapist for other difficulties. Your GP will send a referring letter if you ask him/her. If this is not possible in your area, there may be an Aids Demonstration Centre within reasonable travelling distance. These centres give free advice and are staffed by experienced occupational

110

therapists. To find out if one exists in your area, contact either your local hospital, social services department or health centre.

Social Services Department (for community based nurses, medical social workers, physiotherapists and occupational therapists).

Look in your local Yellow Pages but don't forget that you *must* get your GP to refer you.